ALL YOU NEEDLE
TO KNOW

All you Needle to Know

By Nita Lemonia McHugh

© 2025 by Nita Lemonia McHugh

Published by. Nita Lemonia McHugh

Published in 2025

First Edition

ISBN: 978-0-646-71510-0

Imprint: Independently published

Cover Design by hcjart.com.au | stock glove image by freepik

Any resemblance to actual events, locales, or persons, living or dead, is entirely coincidental.

Dedications

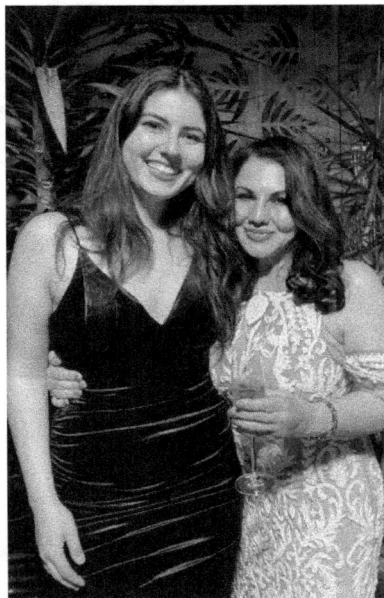

This book is dedicated to my daughter, Antonia, whose patience, curiosity, and sharp wit have been a constant source of inspiration. She spent countless hours in my clinic's waiting room, diligently doing her homework, chatting with clients, and even turning school show-and-tell into a lesson on the differences between fillers and Botox. Her keen eye and clever mind gave this book its perfect title, All You NEEDLE to Know.

Antonia, thank you for growing up alongside my passion and for always believing in the work I do. This book, in many ways, is as much yours as it is mine.

To Dr. Soo-Keat Lim, Your unwavering support and belief in my abilities have been instrumental in shaping my journey. Your mentorship has not only enhanced my professional growth but has also profoundly influenced my personal development. I am deeply grateful for your guidance, which has been a cornerstone in my achievements.

Thank you for believing in me and guiding me at the very beginning of my aesthetic journey. Together, we founded Rejuven8 Cosmetic Clinic—one of the first of its kind in Western Sydney—and your unwavering support, kindness, and faith in my abilities made all the difference.

A true gentleman, a pioneer in liposculpture, and a past president of the ACCS, your generosity with knowledge and your humility in treating every patient equally—no matter their walk of life—continues to inspire me.

With deepest appreciation,

Nita Lemonia McHugh

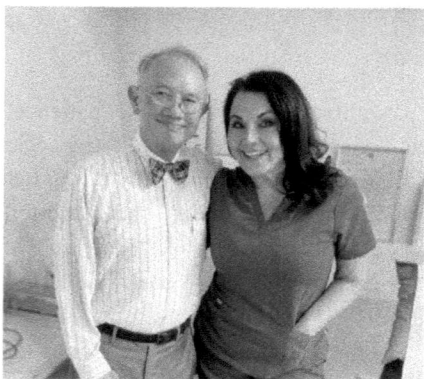

Esteemed Cosmetic Physician , former President of the ACCS. Dr Soo-Keat Lim . Working together since 1998. We often joke that our working relationship has lasted more than most marriages!

"To my son, Mathew whose courage and determination inspire me daily. Your strength in overcoming adversity is a testament to the human spirit."

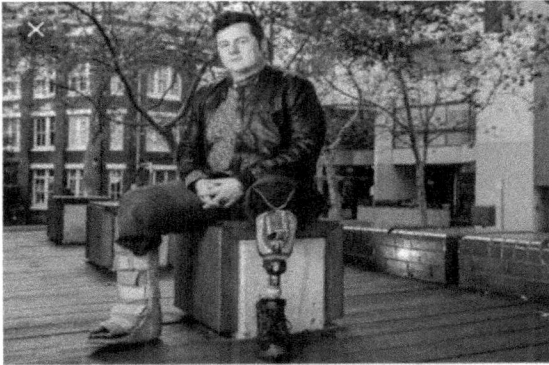

Daily Telegraph

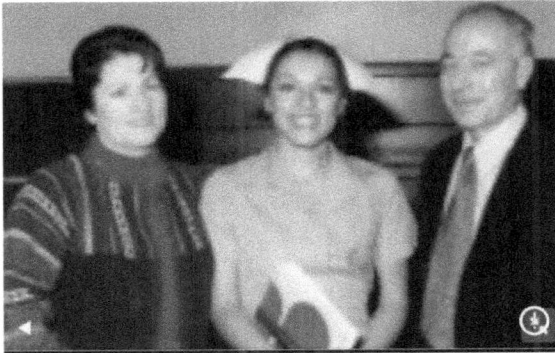

To my dear departed parents. Hope I have made you proud. Here I am as a registered nurse in 1974 receiving the Superintendent Proficiency award , with my parents.

Author's Note

This book is not a textbook. It is a collection of my thoughts, knowledge, and insights gathered over the course of my career in aesthetics. It's my way of sharing the lessons I've learned—the pearls, the pitfalls, and the personal philosophies that have shaped my approach.

It is, in essence, my legacy—offered to newcomers stepping into this field and to educated consumers who want to understand more deeply the treatments they seek.

To my clients: thank you. You made this journey not only meaningful but memorable. We've shared so much more than aesthetic transformations. We've walked through life's milestones together—engagements, weddings, new babies, the heartbreak of loss, divorce, grief. Through all of it, aesthetics became more than skin deep. It became a tool for confidence, resilience, and connection.

With heartfelt gratitude,

Nita McHugh

Registered Nurse, Aesthetic Educator, Cosmetic Injector

Instagram: @nitamchugh_rn

Website: www.nitamchugh.com

Email: cosmeticnurse@outlook.com.

About the Author

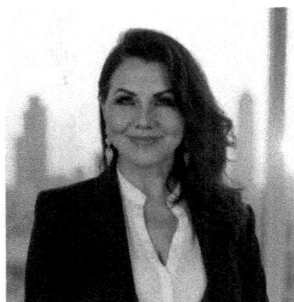

Lemonia Nita McHugh

Nita Lemonia McHugh is a highly experienced Registered Nurse with 50 years in the field, including 30 years dedicated to aesthetics. Her expertise spans across various advanced injectable treatments, with a strong focus on safety, technique, and achieving natural-looking results.

Nita has been a PRP trainer for AMSL and a Radiesse trainer for Merz, sharing her in-depth knowledge with fellow practitioners. She worked alongside esteemed cosmetic physician Dr. Soo Keat Lim for 25 years and has spent the last five years working with Professor Tim Papadopoulos, providing aesthetic services in Western Sydney, Australia.

Passionate about continuous learning, Nita has attended numerous international conferences, company workshops, and advanced training sessions. She further refined her anatomical knowledge by participating in a cadaver hands-on course at King's College London, ensuring her techniques are both safe and precise.

Her commitment to patient safety, cutting-edge techniques, and natural aesthetic outcomes has made her a respected professional in the field of cosmetic injectables.

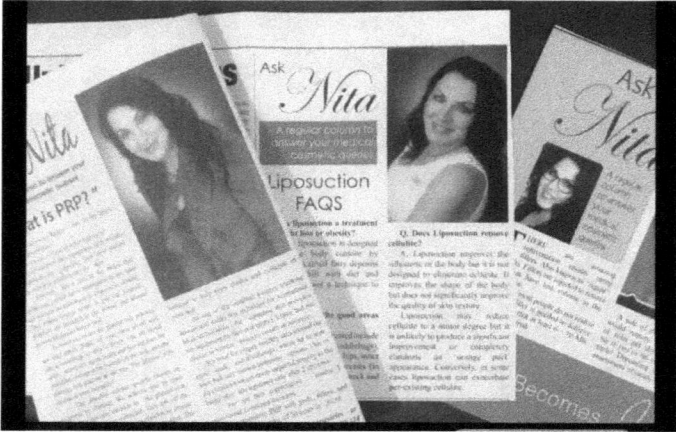

For years, Nita was a regular columnist for Nepean News, writing the popular "Ask Nita" editorial. Through this platform, she educated the Nepean district of Western Sydney about cosmetic injectable procedures and products, helping readers make informed decisions about aesthetic treatments

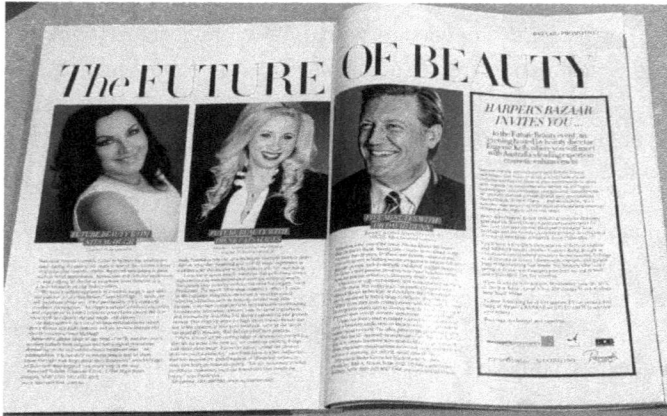

Nita McHugh featured in Harper's Bazaar Magazine July 2012.

ALL YOU NEEDLE TO KNOW

Table of Contents

To my colleagues — pictured and not — thank you for the laughter and support you brought to my aesthetic career.

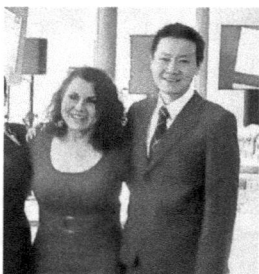

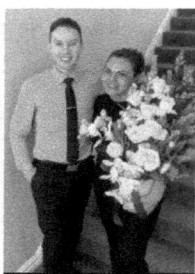

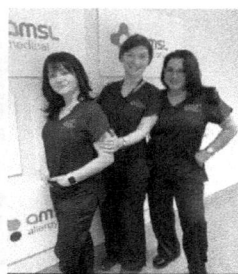

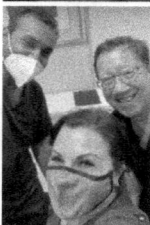

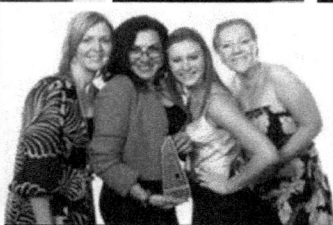

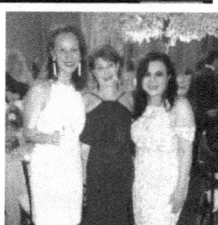

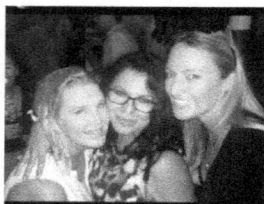

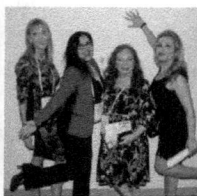

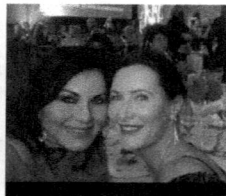

Foreward from A/Prof. Tim Papadopoulos

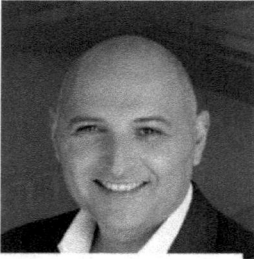

With great pleasure, I introduce "All You NEEDLE to Know," a comprehensive guide to the world of aesthetic injectables written by Nita McHugh, RN. With 50 years of nursing experience and 30 years dedicated to aesthetic medicine, Nita brings unparalleled expertise to this subject. Throughout these pages, she seamlessly blends scientific knowledge with practical wisdom, offering valuable insights for both practitioners and patients. What makes this book exceptional is Nita's ability to demystify complex concepts while maintaining clinical accuracy. Her patient-centred approach shines through in every chapter, emphasising safety, natural results, and ethical practice. From the science of botulinum toxin and dermal fillers to regenerative treatments and emerging technologies, Nita covers the full spectrum of injectable aesthetics with clarity and depth. I have witnessed Nita's dedication to excellence and continuous learning throughout her career. I can attest to her commitment to advancing the field of aesthetic medicine. Her focus on evidence-based practices and holistic patient care exemplifies the highest standards of our profession. This book represents her extensive knowledge and passion for educating others and improving patient outcomes.

"All You NEEDLE to Know" will be an invaluable resource for healthcare professionals seeking to enhance their understanding of aesthetic injectables and patients wanting to make informed treatment decisions. It is a testament to Nita's legacy as a skilled practitioner and a generous educator.

A/Prof. Tim Papadopoulos
BSc, MBBS, MBA, FRACS (Gen), FRACS (Plast), GAICD

Foreward from Dr Bonnie Hawthorne

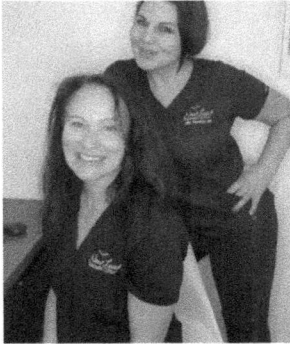

It is an honor to introduce this book, written by someone with a profound understanding of cosmetic injectables and the true essence of beauty. I have been privileged to learn from Nita McHugh, a master of her craft and, in my opinion, a true artist with decades of experience.

Nita possesses a rare gift—the ability to empower individuals to feel confident in their own skin. Her knowledge, skill, and passion shine through in every aspect of her work, and she has successfully shared that wisdom within these pages.

On a personal note, I want to express just how much Nita means to me. She is more than a mentor; she is my teacher, my guide, and my Mama No. 2. Her honesty, talent, and unwavering dedication to her craft are truly inspiring. Every time I watch her work, I am in awe of her unique approach, her meticulous attention to detail, and the care she brings to every procedure. Nita, you are one of a kind—a compassionate healer, a gifted educator, and a guardian angel to those lucky enough to know you. I am incredibly grateful to have you in my life, and I know that readers of this book will gain invaluable insight from your expertise.

Dr. Bonnie Hawthorne
MD MRCS(ENG) DFSRH FRAC GP
Cosmetic Physician

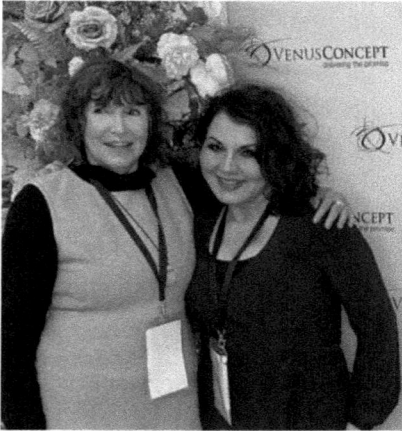

I first met Nita when she attended one of my Paramedical training courses. I was impressed from day one with her professionalism and her desire to work at a high standard, in the cosmetic enhancement industry. Nita, over the years, has made sure that she attended every training available and that her standard of care was always the highest possible.

Her patient interactions were always based on that extremely high knowledge base as well as her desire to do the right thing from a knowledge sharing basis for all who worked for her as well. I feel that Nita's contribution to the cosmetic enhancement industry has been great and will continue to be so for many years to come. This book is another way for Nita to give to the industry she so loves.

Ricky Allen
Beauty Editor Vogue Magazine
Nurse Educator

Preface

Over the past three decades in the aesthetic field, I have dedicated myself to continuous learning and professional development. Attending hundreds of conferences, participating in numerous company trainings, and engaging with a diverse client base have all contributed to a wealth of knowledge and experience that I am eager to share.

In Australia, the Therapeutic Goods Administration (TGA) enforces strict regulations against the advertising of cosmetic injectables. This has highlighted the need for clients to be well-informed and educated when considering aesthetic procedures. It is crucial to choose experienced healthcare professionals and avoid unqualified operators.

I am committed to lifelong learning and encourage consumers to educate themselves thoroughly before embarking on aesthetic treatments. Enhancing one's appearance is not an act of vanity but a form of self-care. Looking refreshed can help individuals feel good, maintain confidence, and continue to engage actively in various aspects of life, whether it's remaining in the workforce or re-entering the dating scene.

My passion lies in natural enhancement and restoring confidence through informed, safe, and effective aesthetic practices.

Welcome to ALL YOU NEEDLE TO KNOW—your essential guide to the world of cosmetic injectables. If you've ever considered an aesthetic treatment but felt overwhelmed by the vast array of options, confusing terminology, or conflicting information, you're not alone. This book is here to simplify the process, answer your questions, and empower you with knowledge so that you can make informed decisions about your skin and overall appearance.

I'm Nita McHugh, a registered nurse since 1978 and an aesthetic nurse for over 30 years. My personal journey into cosmetic injectables began with my own desire to correct my skin and smooth out frown lines. I initially started with medical skin treatments before incorporating injectables into my practice. Having started Botox treatments at age 38, I understand firsthand both the curiosity and concerns that come with aesthetic enhancements. Over the years, I have worked with countless clients who, like you, want to look refreshed and natural—not "overdone" or unrecognisable.

Cosmetic injectables have come a long way from the early days of Botox and dermal fillers. Today, the industry offers a wide range of treatments designed not only to smooth wrinkles but also to enhance facial contours, restore lost volume, and even improve skin quality. However, with more choices comes more confusion. Should you opt for Botox or a filler? What's the difference between hyaluronic acid and biostimulatory injectables? How do you ensure that your treatment results are both safe and effective?

This book will break down everything you need to know, from the science behind injectables to the practicalities of choosing a qualified practitioner. Based in Sydney, Australia, I have witnessed the evolution of this industry and the growing demand for natural, rejuvenating treatments. My goal is to cut through the marketing hype and provide clear, factual, and professional insights, ensuring that you decide with the confidence, to make the best choices for yourself.

Whether you're completely new to the world of injectables or looking to refine your knowledge, ALL YOU NEEDLE TO KNOW will serve as your trusted companion in navigating this exciting and ever-advancing field.

Let's get started on your journey to informed and confident beauty choices!

CHAPTER 1: MY PERSONAL AESTHETIC JOURNEY

At age 35, I became aware of a feature I couldn't ignore my frown lines. I frowned when driving, when thinking, and even while sleeping. It became so habitual that I tried placing a band aid on my forehead at night to prevent the movement. Unfortunately, this only deepened the creases rather than smoothing them.

Then, I discovered Botox. It was a revelation. The ability to relax the muscles responsible for my frown lines transformed my expression and, in many ways, my confidence. Now, 35 years later, my frown has vanished not just because of Botox but also due to behaviour modification. My brain has learned that frowning is unnecessary, and I no longer require frequent treatments.

Exploring Other Aesthetic Enhancements

While Botox was my entry into the world of aesthetics, over the years, I have explored a variety of treatments to maintain and enhance my natural beauty.

Fillers: A Love-Hate Relationship

I have had dermal fillers in my lips and lateral cheeks, enhancing volume and contour. However, because I naturally have a full face, I found that fillers sometimes made me look puffy rather than refreshed. This led me to explore alternative treatments for a more natural result.

Surgical Enhancements: A Delicate Balance

As I aged, my eyes began to show signs of heaviness. To address this, I underwent upper and lower blepharoplasty a subtle yet impactful procedure that rejuvenated my eyes without changing my natural expression. It was one of the best decisions I made, as it restored brightness to my face.

The Shift to Regenerative Aesthetics

In recent years, I have embraced regenerative treatments. Instead of simply filling and plumping, I wanted to stimulate my body's natural collagen production for longer-lasting, authentic results.

Sculptra: I love how Sculptra gradually builds collagen rather than just adding volume. It provides a natural lift and firmness, avoiding the overfilled look fillers sometimes create.

 Radiesse for the Jawline: For a structured, defined jawline, I have found Radiesse to be a game-changer. It provides immediate contour while also stimulating collagen over time.

Annual PRP (Platelet-Rich Plasma) Treatments: I believe in the power of PRP, not just for skin but also for hair rejuvenation. I have it done annually on my face, neck, and scalp to boost collagen, improve texture, and maintain hair thickness.

What Didn't t Work for Me?

Not every treatment suited me, and that's part of the aesthetic journey.

Thread Lifting: I tried it but wasn't impressed. The discomfort and temporary results didn't justify the effort for me. I do believe my face is too heavy for threads. They work well for suitable candidates.

My Commitment to Skin Health

Beyond injectables and regenerative treatments, skin quality has always been a priority for me.

Frequent Skin Treatments: I maintain my skin integrity with regular treatments.

Chemical Peels & Dermapen: To refine texture and stimulate collagen, I incorporate chemical peels and microneedling (Dermapen).

MOXI Laser: This treatment has been a great addition to my regimen, addressing pigmentation and skin tone irregularities while keeping my skin glowing.

Ultherapy: For skin tightening, Ultherapy has been a favourite.It stimulates collagen deep within the skin, keeping it firm and lifted.

Reflections on My Aesthetic Journey

At almost 70, I stand as an example of natural rejuvenation not by chasing trends, but by making informed choices, balancing intervention with prevention, and embracing treatments that work with my natural features rather than against them.

Aesthetic medicine has evolved immensely since I first started my journey, and I have grown with it. My experience has shaped not only how I treat myself but also how I guide my patients. Looking good is not about fighting ageing it's about aging well, gracefully, and confidently.

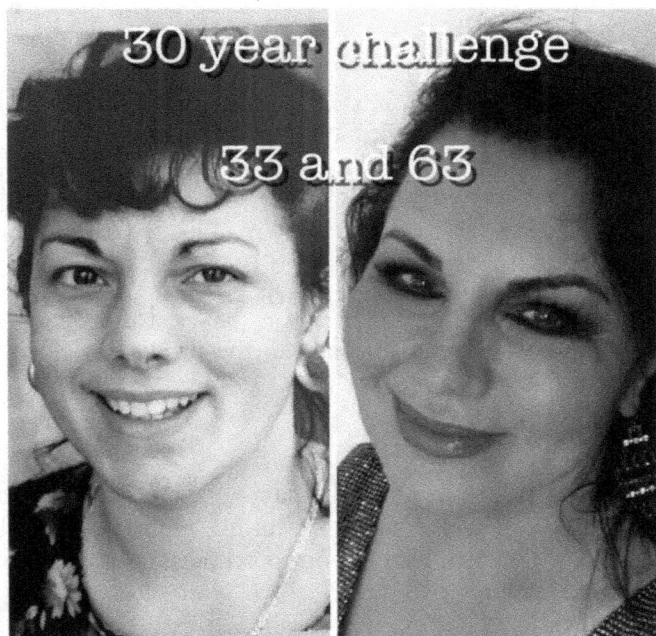

30 year challenge

33 and 63

CHAPTER 2: HOW TO CHOOSE THE RIGHT INJECTOR

The most important decision you will make

When it comes to cosmetic injectables, the product is not the most important factor.

The injector is.

Botulinum toxin, fillers, and biostimulants are just tools. In the right hands, they can create subtle, beautiful, natural results. In the wrong hands, they can lead to poor outcomes, complications, and long-term damage.

Choosing your injector is the single most important decision in your aesthetic journey.

Why the Injector Matters More Than the Product

Many patients ask:

"What brand of filler do you use?"

But a more important question is:

"Who is holding the syringe?"
A skilled injector understands:

- Facial anatomy

- Aging patterns

- Proportions and balance

- Emotional anatomy
- Safety protocols
- Complication management

The same product in different hands can produce:

- Elegant, natural results or
- Overfilled, distorted features

It's not the syringe.

It's the artist.

Types of Injectors: Who Can Perform Treatments?

In Australia and many other countries, cosmetic injectables may be performed by:

- Doctors
- Registered nurses
- Nurse practitioners
- Dentists (in some areas)

Each profession can be competent—but experience and training matter more than the title.

A nurse with 15 years of aesthetic experience may be far more skilled than a doctor who has just completed a weekend course.

What matters most is:

- Experience
- Ongoing education
- Safety knowledge
- Aesthetic eye

The Experience Factor

Cosmetic injecting is both a science and an art.

It takes years to master.

When choosing an injector, ask:

- How many years have you been injecting?
- Do you inject full time or occasionally?
- How often do you attend training or conferences?

Experience teaches:

- How faces age
- How different products behave
- How to avoid complications
- How to manage complications if they occur

An injector who has treated thousands of faces will see things a beginner may miss.

What to Look for in a Good Injector

1. A Natural Aesthetic

Look at their work:

- Do their patients look natural?
- Or do they look overfilled and artificial?

A good injector aims for:

- Balance
- Subtlety

- Harmony
- Age-appropriate results

If all their patients have:

- Overfilled lips
- Frozen foreheads
- Identical faces

…that may not be the right clinic for you.

2. A Proper Consultation

A professional injector will:

- Ask about your medical history
- Discuss your concerns
- Examine your face from different angles
- Explain treatment options
- Set realistic expectations

Red flag:

If the injector asks:

"How many syringes do you want?"
before even looking at your face.

3. They Can Say "No"

This is one of the most important signs of a good injector.

A responsible practitioner will:

- Refuse unrealistic requests
- Decline unsafe treatments

- Suggest alternatives

If someone is willing to inject anything, anywhere, at any time, just because you asked—that is not safe practice.

4. They Explain Risks and Complications

A skilled injector will:

- Discuss possible side effects
- Explain complications honestly
- Provide written aftercare
- Offer follow-up appointments

They should also have:

- Emergency protocols
- Reversal agents
- Training in complication management

You can ask:

- Do you carry hyaluronidase?
- What do you do if a vessel is blocked?

A confident injector will answer calmly and clearly.

5. A Clean, Professional Environment

The clinic should:

- Be clean and well-organised
- Use sterile, single-use needles
- Have proper medical supplies
- Maintain professional standards

If it feels like a backroom operation, beauty party, or pop-up event, think carefully before proceeding.

Red Flags When Choosing an Injector

Be cautious if you notice:

- Extremely cheap prices
- Constant discount promotions
- No consultation offered
- Pressure to buy packages
- No discussion of risks
- No follow-up offered
- Treatments done in non-medical settings
- Overfilled faces everywhere on their social media

Remember:

If the price seems too good to be true, it usually is.

Cheap work can become very expensive to fix.

Social Media vs. Real Experience

Today, many injectors are judged by:

- Instagram followers
- TikTok videos
- Before-and-after photos

But social media does not always reflect:

- Real skill
- Long-term results
- Complication management
- Ethical practice

Some of the best injectors:

- Have modest social media
- Rely on word-of-mouth
- Have long-term loyal patients

Experience matters more than online popularity.

Questions Every Patient Should Ask

Before treatment, ask:

1. How many years have you been injecting?
2. What training have you completed?
3. Do you carry hyaluronidase?
4. What is your emergency protocol?
5. Do you offer follow-up reviews?

These questions are not rude.

They are responsible.

The Importance of a Treatment Plan

A good injector will not just treat one line or one area.

They will:

- Assess the whole face

- Consider proportions
- Plan long-term results
- Suggest staged treatments if needed

A thoughtful treatment plan leads to:

- Better results
- More natural outcomes
- Fewer complications
- Better value over time

The Cheapest Treatment Is Not the Best Value

Patients often shop around for the lowest price.

But in aesthetics, price often reflects:

- Experience
- Product quality
- Clinic standards
- Time spent in consultation
- Safety protocols

Poor treatments may lead to:

- Dissolving filler
- Corrective procedures
- Emotional distress
- Additional costs

In the long run, good work is always better value.

When choosing an injector, trust:

- Experience over hype
- Skill over price
- Natural results over trends
- Professionalism over popularity

The right injector will make you feel:

- Heard
- Respected
- Safe
- Understood

And when the work is done well, people won't say:

"Who did your lips?"
They'll say:

"You look fantastic."
That's the true sign of a great injector.

Chapter 3: What to Expect at the Initial Consultation

Procedure at Consultation: What to Expect

A thorough consultation is essential before any aesthetic treatment to ensure safety, suitability, and optimal results. The clinician will assess your medical history, concerns, and contributing factors before designing a personalized treatment plan.

1. Medical History & Lifestyle Factors

Previous Aesthetic Treatments:

Have you had fillers, Botox, lasers, or skin treatments before?

Any adverse reactions or complications?

Medical Conditions:

Autoimmune disorders (e.g., lupus, rheumatoid arthritis)

Skin conditions (e.g., rosacea, eczema, psoriasis)

Bleeding disorders or clotting issues

Medications & Supplements:

• Blood thinners (Aspirin, Warfarin, Clopidogrel, NSAIDs) → Increase bruising risk

• Steroids or Immunosuppressants → Affect healing & collagen response

• Herbal supplements (Ginkgo, Garlic, Fish Oil) → May cause excessive bleeding

• Accutane (Isotretinoin) → Recent use can impact skin healing

Lifestyle Considerations:

• Smoking & Alcohol Consumption → Affect healing & skin health

• Sun Exposure & Skincare Routine → Important for post-treatment care

2. Blood Health & Bruising Risk

Blood Thinners & Platelet Function

• If taking aspirin, NSAIDs, or anticoagulants, bruising may be more significant.

• Iron levels & anemia may impact healing & collagen stimulation in biostimulants.

Autoimmune & Inflammatory Conditions

• Some conditions can lead to abnormal healing responses or increased risk of reaction.

3. Patient Concerns & Treatment Goals

What are your concerns?

• Volume loss? Wrinkles? Skin laxity? Hyperpigmentation?

• Are there specific areas you want to improve?

What results are you expecting?

• Immediate vs. long-term effects?

• Natural results vs. significant enhancement?

Are you preparing for an event?

• Some treatments require downtime, so planning ahead is crucial.

4. Clinical Examination: Identifying the Root Cause of Concerns

Volume Loss or Laxity? → Is it due to fat loss, skin thinning, or bone resorption?

Wrinkles & Fine Lines? → Are they static (from collagen loss) or dynamic (from muscle movement)?

Skin Texture & Pigmentation? → Sun damage, inflammation, or post-inflammatory hyperpigmentation?

5. Skin & Blood Vessel Examination: Minimizing Risks

Skin Thinners:

• Is the skin thin, fragile, or atrophic?

• Can the chosen treatment be safely administered without excessive trauma?

Herpes Simplex (Cold Sores on Lips):

• If treating the lips, history of cold sores (HSV-1) is important.

• Pre-treatment antiviral medication (e.g., Acyclovir or Valacyclovir) may be prescribed to prevent an outbreak.

Final Steps Before Proceeding with Treatment

•Explain the Treatment Plan & Expected Outcomes

•Discuss Risks, Side Effects & Aftercare

• Obtain Informed Consent

Doctor to confirm and approve treatment plan and script for the treating Cosmetic RN.

A thorough consultation ensures patient safety, personalized care, and optimal results for every treatment.

The initial consultation involves a detailed discussion of concerns, followed by a comprehensive facial examination. This assessment covers various structural and aesthetic aspects of the face to determine the most effective approach for treatment.

Facial Examination Includes:

• **Bone Structure** – Evaluating the underlying framework that supports facial contours.

• **Deep Fat Pads** – Assessing volume loss that contributes to ageing and changes in facial shape.

• **Muscle Actions** – Observing how facial muscles move and contribute to expressions and wrinkles.

• **Ligaments** – Identifying areas where support has weakened, leading to sagging.

• **Shallow Fat Pads** – Examining surface-level fat that affects facial fullness and contour.

- **Skin Quality** – Assessing dynamic lines, crepey skin, texture, and overall skin health.

- **Facial Symmetry** – Identify facial asymmetry, as most people have a wider side.

Rather than treating just the surface concerns, the focus is on identifying and addressing the root cause. For example, nasolabial folds (the lines running from the nose to the corners of the mouth) are often not directly filled. Instead, volume loss in the lateral fat pads, cheekbones, and surrounding structures is corrected to restore natural contour and lift, leading to a more balanced and youthful appearance and lessening the depth of the naso labial folds.

This holistic approach ensures a personalised treatment plan that enhances facial harmony while maintaining a natural look

CHAPTER 4: THE PSYCHOLOGY BEHIND COSMETIC TREATMENTS

Procedure at Consultation: What to Expect

Treating the person, not just the face

Cosmetic treatments are often spoken about in terms of muscles, volume, collagen, and skin quality. But after more than 30 years in the treatment room, I can tell you this:

People don't come in because of wrinkles.

They come in because of how those wrinkles make them feel.

Behind every request for Botox, filler, or a skin treatment is a story. Sometimes it's about confidence. Sometimes it's about loss, stress, divorce, illness, or simply the shock of looking in the mirror and not recognising yourself anymore.

Understanding the psychology behind cosmetic treatments is just as important as understanding the anatomy of the face.

Why People Really Seek Treatment

Most patients don't say:

"I want my corrugator muscles weakened."
They say:

- "I look tired all the time."

- "I look angry, even when I'm not."

- "I don't feel like myself anymore."

- "I just want to look fresher."

Cosmetic treatments are rarely about vanity alone. They are often about:

- Restoring confidence
- Matching the outside to how someone feels inside
- Regaining control during a difficult time
- Looking more professional at work
- Feeling attractive again after divorce or illness

Many patients are going through life transitions:

- Menopause
- Retirement
- Divorce
- Career changes
- Children leaving home
- Illness or recovery

When the face starts to change, it can feel like a loss of identity.

The Mirror and the Mind

The face is deeply connected to our sense of self.

It is:

- How we recognise ourselves
- How others respond to us
- How we express emotions
- How we communicate

When someone looks in the mirror and sees:

- Sagging skin

- Deep lines

- Hollow eyes

- A tired or sad expression

…it can affect their mood, confidence, and even how they behave socially.

I've had patients say:

- "I stopped going out."

- "I don't like photos anymore."

- "I feel invisible."

Small, subtle treatments can sometimes create a powerful emotional shift.

Not because the person looks like someone else—

but because they start to look like themselves again.

Confidence vs. Insecurity

There is a big difference between:

Healthy cosmetic motivation And unhealthy psychological drivers

Healthy motivations

- Wanting to look fresher

- Wanting subtle improvement

- Accepting aging but wanting support

- Realistic expectations

These patients are usually:

- Calm
- Open to advice
- Happy with natural results

Unhealthy motivations

- Obsessive focus on tiny flaws
- Unrealistic expectations
- Wanting to look like a celebrity or filter
- Constant dissatisfaction with results

These patients may:

- Doctor shop
- Demand more product
- Never feel satisfied
- Blame the injector for emotional issues

This is where psychology becomes critical.

Body Dysmorphic Tendencies

Body Dysmorphic Disorder (BDD) is a psychological condition where a person becomes obsessed with perceived flaws that others may not even notice.

Signs may include:

- Constant mirror checking
- Extreme dissatisfaction with appearance
- Repeated cosmetic treatments without satisfaction
- Fixation on one small area

- Unrealistic expectations

These patients are not good candidates for cosmetic treatment.

No amount of filler or Botox will solve a psychological issue.

An ethical injector must sometimes say:

"I don't think treatment is the right solution for you at this time."

This can be uncomfortable—but it is the right thing to do.

The Emotional Consultation

A good consultation is not just about the face.

It is about:

- Listening

- Observing

- Understanding the patient's emotional state

Sometimes the real issue isn't the wrinkle.

It's what the wrinkle represents.

For example:

A patient says:

"I hate these lines around my mouth."

But as the consultation unfolds, you discover:

- She has recently gone through a divorce

- She feels unattractive

- She hasn't dated in years

The treatment becomes more than a cosmetic fix.

It becomes part of a confidence rebuilding process.

The Danger of Social Media and Filters

We now live in a world of:

- Filters

- Editing apps

- AI-enhanced images

- Unrealistic beauty standards

Many patients bring in filtered photos and say:

"I want to look like this."
But those images:

- Are not real

- Have altered proportions

- Remove natural facial movement

- Erase pores and texture

This creates a dangerous gap between:

Reality and expectation

An experienced injector helps patients understand:

- What is achievable

- What is natural

- What suits their face

The Role of the Injector: Technician or Guide?

A good injector is not just a technician.

They are part:

- Artist

- Clinician

- Listener

- Guide

Your injector should:

- Educate you

- Set realistic expectations

- Say no when necessary

- Recommend what is appropriate, not just what is requested

Sometimes the best treatment is:

- Less product

- A different approach

- Or no treatment at all

Midlife, Hormones, and Identity

Many cosmetic patients are in midlife, especially women.

This stage often includes:

- Hormonal changes

- Menopause

- Children leaving home

- Career transitions

- Relationship changes

The face changes at the same time life is changing.

This can create a feeling of:

- Loss of youth
- Loss of identity
- Loss of attractiveness

Cosmetic treatments, when done well, can:

- Restore confidence
- Improve self-image
- Help patients feel more like themselves again

The Power of Subtle Change

Some of the most emotional moments in my career have not come from dramatic transformations, but from very small ones.

A patient looks in the mirror after a subtle treatment and says:

"Oh… I look like me again."
That moment is not about vanity.

It's about recognition, relief, and confidence.

When to Say No

One of the most important skills in aesthetic medicine is knowing when not to treat.

Reasons to say no:

- Unrealistic expectations
- Emotional instability
- Body dysmorphic tendencies
- Pressure from partners or friends
- Very young patients seeking unnecessary treatment

Ethical practice is not about selling syringes.

It is about protecting the patient.

Cosmetic Treatments and Self-Worth

Cosmetic treatments should never be used as a substitute for:

- Self-esteem
- Emotional healing
- Relationship issues
- Mental health support

They can:

- Enhance confidence
- Improve appearance
- Support self-image

But they are not a cure for deeper emotional wounds.

Before having any cosmetic treatment, ask yourself:

- Am I doing this for me, or for someone else?
- Do I want to look fresher, or completely different?
- Are my expectations realistic?
- Would a subtle improvement make me happy?

The best cosmetic treatments are the ones that make people say:

"You look well."
"You look rested."
"You look happy."
Not:

"What have you had done?"
Because the true goal of aesthetics is not to change who you are—

it's to help you feel comfortable in your own skin.

CHAPTER 5: EMOTIONAL ANATOMY OF THE FACE

In aesthetic medicine, we are trained to study anatomy—muscles, fat pads, ligaments, and bone structure. We learn where to inject, how deep to go, and how many units or millilitres to use.

But after more than 30 years in the treatment room, I've come to understand something even more important:

Every face has an emotional anatomy.

Behind every wrinkle, every hollow, every request for Botox or filler, there is often a feeling, a story, or a life transition. People don't come in because of muscles or collagen loss. They come in because of how their face makes them feel.

If you truly want to understand cosmetic treatments, you must understand not just the physical anatomy of the face—but the emotional anatomy as well.

What Is Emotional Anatomy?

Emotional anatomy is the idea that different areas of the face are connected to certain expressions, moods, and psychological messages.

Over time, the face can begin to reflect:

- Stress

- Fatigue

- Sadness

- Anger

- Worry

- Loss

- Life experiences

Sometimes these expressions become permanent, even when the person no longer feels that way.

For example:

- Frown lines can make someone look angry.

- Drooping mouth corners can create a sad appearance.

- Hollow under-eyes can make someone look exhausted.

- Heavy brows can give a stern or tired look.

Patients often say:

- "I look angry all the time."

- "People keep asking if I'm tired."

- "I look sad in photos."

What they are noticing is not just aging.

They are noticing changes in their emotional anatomy.

The Emotional Map of the Face

Over decades of practice, certain patterns appear again and again. Different areas of the face tend to communicate different emotional signals.

The Forehead and Frown Area

Emotional message:

Worry, anger, stress, seriousness

Deep frown lines between the brows can give the impression of:

- Irritation

- Tension

- Harshness

- Disapproval

Many patients say:

"I don't feel angry, but I look angry."
Softening this area with toxin can:

- Create a more relaxed expression

- Make the face appear kinder and more approachable

The Eyes and Tear Trough

Emotional message:

Fatigue, sadness, exhaustion

Hollow or dark under-eyes often create:

- A tired appearance

- A sad or worn-out look

- The impression of poor health or stress

Patients often say:

"No matter how much I sleep, I still look tired."
Treatments in this area, when done correctly, can:

- Restore brightness

- Soften the tired appearance

- Improve overall facial harmony

The Midface and Cheeks

Emotional message:

Youthfulness, vitality, happiness

Full, lifted cheeks are associated with:

- Youth

- Energy

- Positivity

As volume is lost in the midface:

- The face can look flat

- The mouth corners may drop

- The overall expression may look sad or heavy

Restoring subtle cheek support can:

- Lift the lower face

- Improve the emotional expression

- Make the face appear more vibrant

The Mouth and Lower Face

Emotional message:

Sadness, disappointment, ageing

Drooping mouth corners and marionette lines can create:

- A sad or bitter expression

- A tired or aged appearance

- The impression of unhappiness

Patients often say:

"I look miserable, even when I'm in a good mood."

Soft, careful treatments in this area can:

- Lift the corners of the mouth
- Soften harsh lines
- Restore a neutral or gentle expression

The Jawline and Neck

Emotional message:

Strength, confidence, structure

A well-defined jawline is associated with:

- Confidence
- Youth
- Strength
- Vitality

As the jawline softens:

- The face can appear heavier 'jowled'
- The expression may seem tired or less defined

Subtle structural treatments can:

- Restore definition
- Improve facial balance
- Create a more confident profile

Why People Really Seek Treatment

Patients rarely say:

"I want to correct my nasolabial fold."
Instead, they say:

- "I look tired."

- "I look angry."

- "I don't feel like myself anymore."

- "I just want to look fresher."

Cosmetic treatments are often about:

- Restoring confidence

- Matching the outside to how someone feels inside

- Regaining control during a life transition

- Feeling attractive again after illness, divorce, or stress

Many patients come in during periods of change:

- Menopause

- Retirement

- Career transitions

- Relationship breakdowns

- Health challenges

When the face changes at the same time life is changing, it can feel like a loss of identity.

The Mirror and Self-Perception

The face is deeply tied to self-image.

It is:

- How we recognise ourselves

- How we communicate emotions

- How others respond to us

When someone looks in the mirror and sees:

- Deep lines
- Hollow eyes
- Sagging skin
- A tired or sad expression

…it can affect:

- Confidence
- Mood
- Social interactions
- Professional presence

A small, subtle treatment can sometimes create a powerful emotional shift—not because the person looks different, but because they look like themselves again.

Healthy Motivation vs. Emotional Red Flags

Not all cosmetic motivations are healthy.

Healthy motivations

- Wanting to look fresher
- Accepting aging but wanting support
- Realistic expectations
- Desire for subtle improvement

Emotional red flags

- Obsession with tiny flaws
- Wanting to look like a celebrity or filter

- Constant dissatisfaction

- Repeated treatments with no happiness

These patients may need emotional support, not more filler.

The Role of the Injector: Guardian of the Face

A skilled injector is not just a technician.

They are also:

- A listener

- An observer

- A guide

- An ethical decision-maker

They must assess:

- The physical anatomy

- The emotional anatomy

- The patient's expectations

- The psychological readiness for treatment

Sometimes the most professional decision is to say:

"I don't think treatment is right for you at this time."

The Power of Subtle Change

Some of the most meaningful moments in aesthetic practice come from very small changes.

A patient looks in the mirror and says:

"I look like me again."

That moment is not about vanity.

It is about recognition, relief, and confidence.

Before any cosmetic treatment, ask yourself:

- Am I doing this for me?

- Do I want to look fresher or completely different?

- Are my expectations realistic?

- Would a subtle improvement make me happy?

The best cosmetic treatments are the ones that make people say:

"You look well."
"You look rested."
"You look happy."
Not:

"What have you had done?"
Because the true goal of aesthetics is not to change who you are—

it is to help your outer face reflect your inner self.

That is the art of working with both the physical anatomy and the emotional anatomy of the face.

CHAPTER 6: COSMETIC PROCEDURES AMONGST DIFFERENT AGE GROUPS

As the field of aesthetic medicine evolves, so does our understanding of how different age groups approach cosmetic procedures. The goals of treatment vary depending on the natural aging process, lifestyle factors, and individual aesthetic desires. In this chapter, we explore the nuances of cosmetic procedures across different age groups:

Ages 18-30: Beautification & Prevention

At this stage, youthful skin, collagen production, and elasticity are at their peak. However, early preventative treatments and subtle enhancements are popular in this group, particularly influenced by social media, celebrity culture, and personal aesthetics.

Common Procedure

Neurotoxin (Botox, Dysport, Xeomin): Preventative treatment to reduce excessive muscle movement and delay wrinkle formation (e.g., forehead lines, frown lines, crow's feet).

Lip Enhancement (Dermal Fillers): Subtle volume enhancement, hydration, and definition without overfilling.

Jawline & Chin Contouring: Using fillers to enhance facial symmetry and definition, particularly in profile balancing.

Cheekbone Enhancement: Adding structure and contour with HA (hyaluronic acid) fillers.

Hydrating & Skin Treatments: PRP, skin boosters, microneedling, and mesotherapy to maintain skin health.

Chemical Peels & Laser Treatments: Addressing early pigmentation, acne scars, and overall skin clarity.

Preventative Skincare: Regimen Medical-grade skincare with SPF, retinol, and antioxidants to slow aging.

Goal: Subtle enhancements, maintaining youthful features, and preventing early signs of aging.

Ages 30-45: Beautification, Prevention, & Correction

This age group focuses on both prevention and correction as collagen production begins to slow. Fine lines may start appearing, and volume loss becomes noticeable in some areas.

Common Procedures

Botox & Neurotoxin :Continued use for both prevention and correction of expression lines.

Fillers for Volume Loss : Mid-face (cheeks) to maintain youthful contours, tear troughs to reduce tired appearance.

Nasolabial Fold & Marionette Line Correction :Subtle filler to soften early signs of aging.

Skin Tightening Procedures: Radiofrequency (RF) micro needling, ultrasound therapy (Ultherapy), or fractional lasers.

Jawline & Lower Face Refinement: Addressing early sagging with fillers, collagen-stimulating injectables like Sculptra or Radiesse.

Lip & Chin Enhancements: Maintaining natural proportions and restoring volume.

PRP & Biostimulators : Encouraging collagen production for long-term anti-aging benefits.

Goal: Maintaining youthful appearance while addressing early signs of aging and structural support.

Ages 45-65: Beautification, Prevention, Correction & Restoring

During this phase, skin elasticity reduces, facial fat loss accelerates, and deeper wrinkles form. The aim shifts toward rejuvenation, lifting, and maintaining structural integrity.

Common Procedures

Advanced Botox Application: Smoothing dynamic wrinkles while maintaining natural expression.

Full-Face Filler Approach : Strategic placement in temples, cheeks, jawline, and chin to restore lost volume.

Collagen-Stimulating Injectables (Sculptra, Radiesse) Biostimulatory fillers that work with the body's natural collagen production.

Thread Lifts: For mild lifting effects without surgery.

Skin Resurfacing Treatments : CO_2 lasers, RF micro needling, and deep chemical peels for improved texture.

Non-Surgical Neck & Jawline Tightening: HIFU, RF treatments, or submental fat dissolving injections.

PRP & Exosomes for Hair & Skin Regeneration: Addressing hair thinning and skin laxity.

Goal: Restoring lost volume, correcting deeper wrinkles, and maintaining a refreshed appearance.

Ages 65-85: Beautification (Age-Appropriate), Prevention, Correction, Restoring & Rejuvenation

In this age group, the emphasis is on enhancing natural beauty while respecting the aging process. Treatments should focus on softening lines, maintaining hydration, and restoring facial balance rather than drastic changes.

Common Procedures

Botox for Softening Lines :Light doses to avoid an overdone look.

Strategic Fillers for Facial Harmony . Gentle volumization of the cheeks, lips, and perioral area for a natural result.

Skin Hydration & Revitalization :PRP, mesotherapy, skin boosters to improve elasticity and hydration.

RF & Ultrasound Skin Tightening : Non-invasive treatments for subtle lifting effects.

Fat Transfer & Biostimulators :Long-lasting volume restoration using the body's own fat or collagen-stimulating injectables.

Gentle Laser & Light Treatments :For pigmentation, texture, and improving skin tone.

Goal: Age-appropriate rejuvenation, enhancing skin health, and maintaining facial harmony.

Conclusion

Cosmetic procedures should always be tailored to the individual's age, lifestyle, genetics, and personal goals. Understanding how aesthetic interventions evolve across different life stages ensures natural-looking, effective, and ethical treatments.

By approaching each decade with a strategic, science-backed plan, practitioners can deliver results that honour and enhance natural beauty at every age.

CHAPTER 7: MALE FACE

Why Male Aesthetics Require a Different Approach

When it comes to aesthetic treatments like dermal fillers and biostimulators, men require a completely different technique compared to women. The goal is not to feminize but rather to enhance masculinity, restore volume, and maintain a natural, structured appearance.

Key Differences Between Male & Female Faces

Men and women have fundamental anatomical differences in bone structure, fat distribution, and skin thickness, which affect how aging occurs and how fillers should be used.

Facial Features

Male	Female
Cheek Shape Flatter, wider, and less projection	More anterior projection, apple cheeks
Jawline Square, well-defined, strong mandibular angle	More V-shaped, softer transitions
Chin Broader, more horizontal Pointier	more heart-shaped
Skin Thickness Thicker, oilier, more sebaceous glands	Thinner, drier
Brow Position Flatter, more horizontal	Higher arch, softer curve

A mistake often made in male aesthetics is injecting fillers the same way as in women, leading to rounded cheeks, overly projected lips, and a feminized look.

How the Male Face Ages

As men age, they experience:

1. **Bone Resorption**: Loss of volume in the midface, jaw, and chin, causing a weaker jawline and flatter features.

2. **Fat Redistribution**: The loss of deep fat and drooping of superficial fat, creating nasolabial folds, marionette lines, and jowls.

3. **Skin Laxity & Collagen Loss**: Reduction in collagen & elastin, leading to sagging and wrinkles.

4. **Hollowing of Temples & Under Eyes** Giving a tired, sunken look.

Men ageing is more skeletal than soft tissue-driven, meaning strategic structural support is key, rather than excessive volume.

Treatment Approach for Males (Fillers & Biostimulators)

The goal is to restore lost volume while maintaining masculinity.

Key areas for male treatment:

A. Jawline & Chin Enhancement

Define the jawline without excessive width.

Strengthen the mandibular angle and chin projection for a masculine profile.

Products: Radiesse (for structure), Volux, or Ellanse.

Technique: Linear placement along the mandible for a sharp, structured jawline.

B. Midface Rejuvenation (WITHOUT Feminization)

Avoid high, anterior cheek filler to prevent a cheekbone lift look.

Instead, support midface structure with lateral cheek and zygomatic injections.

Products: Sculptra, Radiesse (to stimulate collagen & avoid overfilling).

Technique: Deep placement on bone, avoiding apple cheek projection.

C. Temple & Tear Trough Correction

Hollow temples can age a man's face significantly.

Subtle tear trough correction can refresh the eyes without feminization.

Products: Restylane, Sculptra, or Radiesse in small amounts.

Technique: Low-volume correction, ensuring the face still looks rugged.

D. Forehead & Brow Masculinization

Avoid excessive brow lifting, which can look unnatural.

For frontal bossing, strategic PCL or PLLA fillers can strengthen the brow.

Products: GOURI (for skin tightening),Elanse (for volume).

Choosing the Right Product: Filler vs. Biostimulator?

Features	Hyaluronic Acid	Biostimulators
Longevity	6-18 months	12-36 months
Effect	Immediate	Gradual improvement
Best for	Quick volume	contouring Collagen stimulation ,long-term support
Risk of Overfilling	Yes (if overused)	No, as it gradually builds tissue
Best choice for men		Biostimulators like Radiesse or Sculptra often work better for men because they provide natural volume & structure without puffiness.

Conclusion: The Key to Natural-Looking Male Aesthetics

Avoid feminization by respecting male anatomy (no overfilled cheeks).

Use structural fillers for jawline, chin, and brow enhancement.

(Radiesse, Sculptra, GOURI) are preferred for natural collagen-building.

Subtle corrections to temples, under-eyes, and midface rejuvenation should be done with caution.

CHAPTER 8: GENDER AFFIRMING AESTHETICS – ALIGNING FEATURES WITH IDENTITY

Aesthetic medicine plays a powerful role in helping individuals express their true selves. For many, this means aligning outward features with an inner sense of identity—whether through softening, defining, or harmonising specific areas of the face and body.

Gender affirming aesthetics is not about adhering to binary standards, but rather about supporting each person's journey with precision, respect, and artistry.

For Those Seeking More Feminine Features

Many individuals who wish to present more femininely may desire softness, roundness, and harmony in their facial features. Common aesthetic goals include:

- Forehead and Brows: Creating a smoother, more open look. Botox can lift the brows to create a gentle arch and a more relaxed upper face.

- Cheeks: Adding volume to the midface with fillers creates a rounder, youthful contour.

- Lips: Enhancing volume and definition for a fuller, heart-shaped appearance using hyaluronic acid fillers.

- Chin and Jawline: Softening a square jaw or subtly tapering the chin using filler and/or masseter Botox to reduce width and create a V-shape.

- Nose: Refining nasal contours with dermal filler to create a softer profile.

- Voice-related areas: While surgical procedures address vocal resonance, aesthetic treatments like neck tightening or chin reshaping can complement vocal transition.

For Those Seeking More Masculine Features

Those desiring a more masculine appearance often seek structure, strength, and angularity in the face. Goals may include:

- Brow and Forehead: Lowering or flattening the brow arch using Botox to create a more structured, assertive look.

- Jawline: Enhancing jaw definition with structural fillers like Radiesse or high-density HA fillers to square and widen the lower face.

- Chin: Augmenting projection and width to support a strong, balanced profile.

- Cheeks: Enhancing bone structure with subtle volume to create flatter, angular contours.

- Nose: Strengthening the nasal bridge or defining the tip with non-surgical rhinoplasty.

Skin Concerns in Gender Affirming Aesthetics

Skin plays a crucial role in gender presentation. Hormonal therapy, shaving, and stress can all affect skin health. Common concerns include:

- Acne: Hormonal shifts may trigger breakouts, especially in early transition. Treatments may include salicylic acid, LED therapy, or medical-grade skincare.

- Facial Hair or Shadow: Laser hair removal, electrolysis, or pigment-correcting peels can help reduce beard shadow or excess facial hair.

- Skin Texture: Softening and smoothing the skin with PRP, microneedling, or skin boosters (like NCTF or Volite) helps enhance overall luminosity.

- Pigmentation: Hormonal changes can also trigger melasma or uneven tone; brightening agents or gentle peels can support clear, radiant skin.

- Pore Size and Oiliness: Especially relevant in testosterone therapy. Resurfacing lasers or tailored skincare can reduce excess oil and visible pores.

A Tailored Approach to Identity

Each individual has a unique vision for how they want to look and feel. Practitioners must ask thoughtful, open-ended questions such as:

"What features would you like to enhance or soften?"

"Is there a particular look or feeling you want to achieve?"

The focus should always remain on authentic expression, safety, and emotional well-being. The injector becomes not just a technician, but a partner in transformation—one who listens without assumption and acts with both skill and compassion.

CHAPTER 9: THE BONE BENEATH THE BEAUTY

When we think about aging, we often focus on the skin—wrinkles, sagging, volume loss. But what if I told you that the true culprit behind an aging face is something you don't see? The bones of your skull.

Yes, just like the rest of your body, your skull changes over time. It shrinks, shifts, and resorbs (meaning the body breaks it down and reabsorbs it). This isn't just a random process—it's nature's way of recycling materials. But when it happens in the face, it dramatically affects how we look.

Let's break it down by age.

The Youthful Skull (Teens to Early 30s)

In our younger years, the skull is strong, structured, and proportionate. The eye sockets are relatively smaller, the cheekbones are well-defined, and the jawline is sharp and prominent.

The bone structure acts as a sturdy frame that keeps the soft tissues, like skin and fat, lifted and taut—like a queen-sized quilt perfectly placed on a queen-sized bed. Everything is in balance.

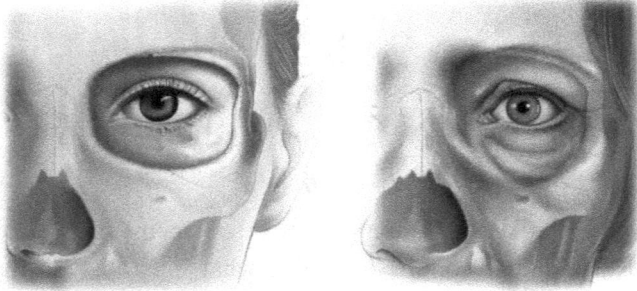

Orbital aging. The superomedial and inferolateral aspects of the orbit have the greatest tendency to resorb. This contributes to the stigmata of periorbital aging such as increased prominence of the medial fat pad, elevation of the medial brow, and langthening of the lid cheek junction.

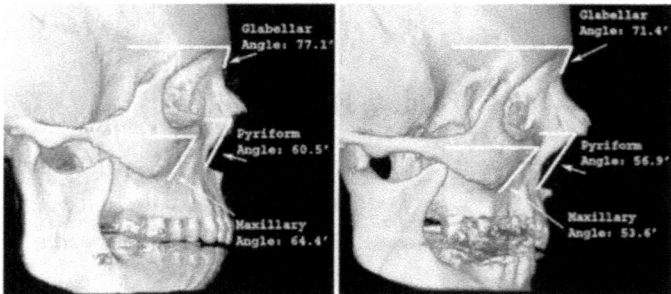

The piriform (piriform angle) and the maxilla (maxillary angle) significantly recede with aging, from youth (left) to old age (right)

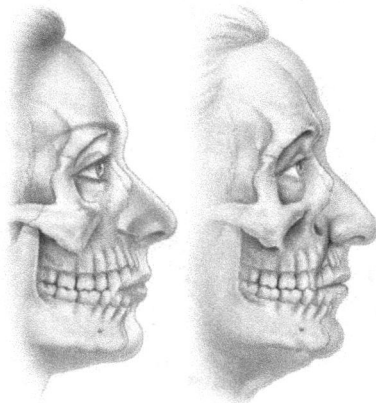

The Loss of bone in the pyriform area weakens the support of the lateral crura. Deepening of the maxilla results in posterior positioning of the nasolabial crease and adjacent upper lip.

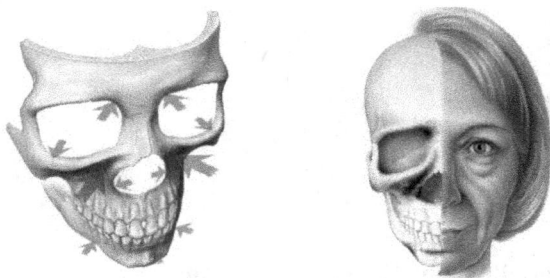

(image left) Arrows indicate the areas of the facial skeleton susceptible to resorption with aging. The size of the arrow correlates with the amount of resorption.

(Image right) The Darker areas are those of the greatest bone loss. The stigmata of aging , manifested by the facial soft tissues, corresponds with the areas of weakened skeletal support.

The Skull : Age related Morphological changes of the Skull

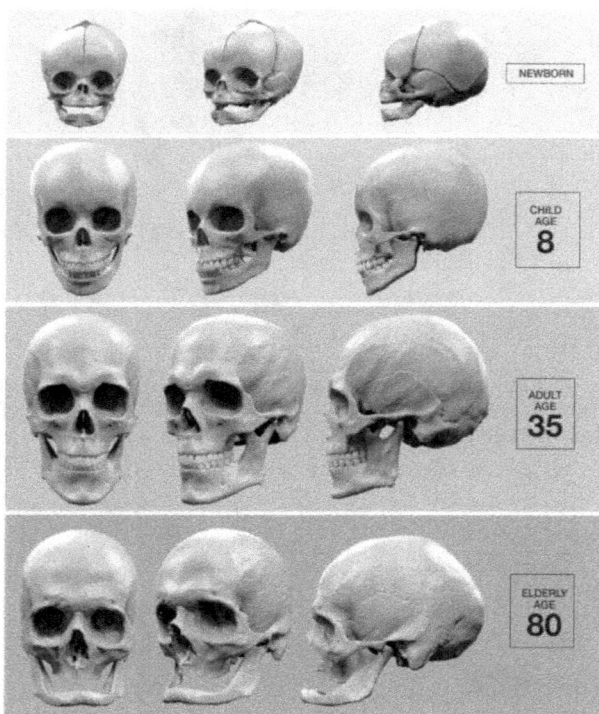

The 30s and 40s: The Beginning of Bone Loss

As we enter our 30s, bone resorption subtly begins. The orbits (eye sockets) start to enlarge, causing the eyes to appear more sunken. The maxilla (midface bone) recedes slightly, making the cheeks look flatter. The jawbone loses density, softening the once-defined jawline.

The chin and mouth area also start to change. The bone supporting the lips recedes, which can make the mouth appear smaller and less structured. This contributes to the development of marionette lines (the lines running from the corners of the mouth downward) and a less defined chin.

Think of it like slightly deflating a balloon—it's not drastic yet, but the structure is starting to weaken.

This is when early signs of aging start to appear, like under-eye hollows, nasolabial folds (smile lines), and a less-defined jawline.

The 50s and Beyond: The Skull Shrinks, The Face Falls

Now the changes become more obvious. The skull has further resorbed, especially in key areas:

• **Eye sockets**: Widen and deepen, making eyes look hollow and tired.

• **Cheekbones**: Flatten further, contributing to sagging skin.

• **Jawbone**: Becomes smaller and less structured, leading to jowls and a receding chin.

• **Nasal bone**: Shrinks slightly, altering the nose shape and making it appear more prominent.

• **Chin and mouth**: The bone surrounding the mouth recedes further, leading to a loss of lip support, increased wrinkling around the mouth, and a downturn of the lips, giving a more aged or sad appearance.

Remember that queen-sized quilt? Imagine putting it on a double bed. Suddenly, it looks oversized and droopy. This is what happens to our face—the skin, muscles, and fat pads no longer fit snugly over the shrinking bone, leading to sagging, folds, and wrinkles.

Why This Matters in Aesthetics

Understanding the role of bone in ageing is crucial when considering cosmetic treatments. Many people think fillers and injectables only address the skin, but the goal is actually to restore the underlying structure.

For example:

•   Temple and cheek fillers help replace lost volume where bone has resorbed, lifting the face naturally.

•   Jawline contouring restores definition lost due to bone shrinkage.

•   Under-eye fillers compensate for the widening of the eye sockets, reducing hollows and shadows.

•   Chin and lip fillers help restore structure and support lost due to bone resorption, improving lip definition and mouth contour.

Modern aesthetics isn't about just chasing lines and wrinkles—it's about rebuilding the foundation.

Conclusion: The Secret to a Youthful Face?

A youthful appearance isn't just about good skin; it's about a strong, structured base. Bone loss is a natural part of ageing, but understanding it allows us to make more informed decisions about aesthetic treatments.

So next time you look in the mirror, remember—it's not just about what's on the surface. The real secret to beauty lies beneath.

Chapter 10: Facial Ligaments: The Framework of Youth

The face is supported by a complex network of ligaments that function like the roots and branches of a tree anchoring soft tissue to bone and maintaining structural integrity. Over time, these ligaments weaken, contributing to sagging, volume loss, and deepening folds. Understanding these ligaments and how they age is crucial in aesthetic medicine, as targeting them with fillers or Platelet-Rich Plasma (PRP) can help restore youthful contours.

What Are Facial Ligaments?

Ligaments are connective tissue structures that either:

1. **True Retaining Ligaments** " These originate from the periosteum (bone covering) and insert into the dermis (skin), acting as strong anchors.

2. **False Retaining Ligaments** (Septal Ligaments) . These do not attach directly to bone but instead suspend soft tissue structures, separating different facial fat compartments.

Key Facial Ligaments and Their Function

1. True Retaining Ligaments (Bone-Anchored)

Orbital Retaining Ligament:Anchors the skin and muscle around the eye socket to the bone, preventing excessive drooping of the eyelids and brows.

Zygomatic (Cheek) Ligament : Extends from the cheekbone (zygomatic arch) to the skin, supporting the midface and nasolabial region.

Masseteric Ligament: Connects the masseter muscle to the skin, defining the jawline and preventing jowl formation.

Mandibular Retaining Ligament :Anchors tissue to the mandible, keeping the lower face firm.

2. False Retaining Ligaments (Soft Tissue Suspensory)

Orbicularis Retaining Ligament.Encircles the eye and blends with surrounding soft tissues, playing a role in eyelid firmness.

Superficial Musculoaponeurotic System (SMAS) Ligaments These septal ligaments form fibrous partitions in the face, segmenting fat compartments and influencing volume distribution.

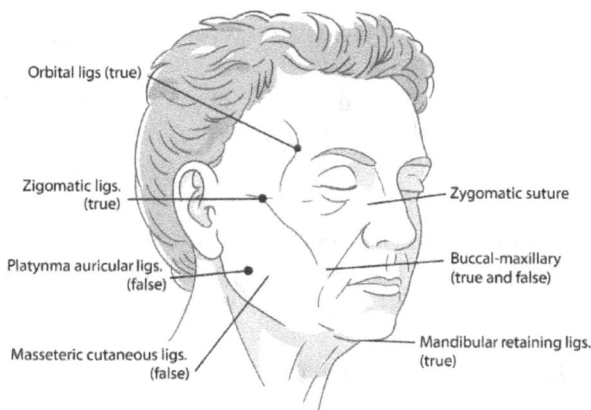

Orbital ligs (true)
Zigomatic ligs. (true)
Platynma auricular ligs. (false)
Masseteric cutaneous ligs. (false)
Zygomatic suture
Buccal-maxillary (true and false)
Mandibular retaining ligs. (true)

How Do Ligaments Age?

With time, facial ligaments undergo:

1. Laxity (Stretching & Weakening) .The collagen fibers in ligaments degrade, causing them to loosen. This leads to ptosis (drooping) of overlying fat and skin.

2. Loss of Fat Volume Support.Fat compartments shrink or descend, exaggerating the appearance of folds and hollows.

3. Bone Resorption .As the underlying bone structure changes (especially in the midface and jawline), ligaments lose their original points of anchorage, exacerbating sagging.

The Aging Effect on Specific Ligaments: Zygomatic Ligament Weakens and deepens naso labial folds.

Mandibular Ligament Weakens jawline and becomes less defined .Jowls Form

Orbital Retaining Ligament:Weakens eyelid skin and skin becomes crepey. Brow Sags

Restoring Ligament Support with PRP and Fillers

To counteract aging-related ligament weakening, PRP (Platelet-Rich Plasma) and dermal fillers can be strategically placed:

1. PRP for Ligament Rejuvenation

PRP contains growth factors that stimulate collagen production and tissue repair. Injecting PRP near weakened ligaments can:

Strengthen the ligamentous structures.

Improve tissue hydration and elasticity.

Delay further degradation of facial support structures.

2. Fillers for Structural Lifting

Fillers can mimic lost fat and volume, repositioning the skin over sagging ligaments. Placing filler under a sagging ligament provides a hammock effect,restoring a more lifted appearance.

Techniques for Ligament-Based Lifting:

Cheek Filler (Zygomatic Ligament Support) Lifts nasolabial folds.

Jawline & Chin Filler (Mandibular Ligament Support) Redefines the jawline, reduces jowls.

Tear Trough & Midface Filler (Orbital & SMAS Support) Reduces hollowing and drooping.

The Tree Analogy: Ligaments as Roots and Fillers as Soil

Imagine ligaments as the roots of a tree, anchoring soft tissue to the bone (trunk). As we age, the roots weaken, and the branches (skin and fat) start to droop. Injecting filler under the ligament is like reinforcing the soil around the tree roots lifting the branches back into place.

Conclusion: A Strategic Approach to Aging Ligament

Understanding the facial ligament system allows aesthetic practitioners to target aging at its source, rather than just filling lines and folds. PRP enhances tissue quality, while fillers placed under sagging ligaments can effectively restore structural support, leading to natural, youthful results.

Chapter 11: Deep Fat Pads in the Face: The Foundation of Volume

The deep fat pads of the face play a crucial role in shaping youthful contours and providing structural support. These fat compartments are located beneath the muscles and help cushion facial movements while maintaining soft, rounded features. However, as we age, these deep fat pads undergo changes that contribute to volume loss, sagging, and facial hollowing. Understanding their anatomy and function is essential for aesthetic interventions such as fillers or fat grafting.

What Are Deep Fat Pads?

Facial fat is divided into two layers:

1. Superficial Fat Pads : Located just beneath the skin, divided into distinct compartments separated by retaining ligaments.

2. Deep Fat Pads : Situated beneath the muscles of facial expression, these pads provide foundational support to the overlying tissues and skin.

Where Are the Deep Fat Pads Located?

The deep fat compartments are primarily found in three key areas of the face:

1. Midface (Cheek Region)

Deep Medial Cheek Fat Pad .The most important deep fat pad, providing volume and projection to the central cheek.

Deep Lateral Cheek Fat Pad :Supports the outer cheek and zygomatic area (cheekbone).

2. Periorbital (Under-Eye) Area

Sub-Orbicularis Oculi Fat (SOOF) Located beneath the orbicularis oculi muscle, crucial for youthful eye contours.

3. Lower Face (Chin and Jawline)

Deep Premaxillary Fat Pad : Provides support beneath the nasolabial folds and upper lip.

Deep Submental Fat Pad : Located under the platysma muscle, affecting the contour of the jawline and neck.

What Is the Purpose of Deep Fat Pads?

1. Structural Support :These pads create foundational volume that holds up the skin and soft tissues.

2. Facial Contouring :They define youthful features, such as full cheeks and a smooth transition from the midface to the lower face.

3. Shock Absorption & Cushioning : Protects muscles and bones from the repetitive movement of facial expressions.

4. Hydration and Elasticity : Fat contains essential lipids that maintain skin hydration and elasticity.

What Happens to Deep Fat Pads as We Age?

1. Volume Loss

Deep fat pads atrophy (shrink) over time, leading to a loss of projection in the cheeks, temples, and under-eye area.

2. Fat Pad Descending & Redistribution

Gravity pulls the fat pads downward. The deep medial cheek fat pad shifts, causing the formation of nasolabial folds and a flattening of the cheeks. The SOOF (under-eye fat pad) descends, resulting in under-eye hollowing and the appearance of eye bags.

3. Bone Resorption and Ligament Weakening

As bone resorbs (shrinks), ligaments loosen, and there is less support for the fat pads. This causes deeper folds and jowling.

4. Changes in the Lower Face

Loss of premaxillary fat leads to upper lip flattening and deeper nasolabial folds. Atrophy of submental fat can contribute to skin laxity under the chin.

Are Deep Fat Pads Located Under Muscle?

Yes, deep fat pads lie beneath the muscles of facial expression, unlike superficial fat pads, which are above them. The SOOF (under-eye fat pad) is under the orbicularis oculi muscle. The deep medial cheek fat pad is under the levator muscles of the midface.

The premaxillary and submental fats are beneath the platysma muscle in the lower face. This positioning makes deep fat pads more resistant to aging than superficial fat, but once volume loss begins, the effects are more pronounced.

Facial nerves :

Facial nerves primarily run beneath deep fat pads, meaning fat acts as a protective cushion for nerve branches. The infraorbital nerve runs beneath the deep medial cheek fat pad, providing sensation to the midface.

The buccal branches of the facial nerve pass through the deep lateral cheek fat, affecting muscle movement. The marginal mandibular nerve runs under the submental and lower cheek fat, controlling lower facial expressions. This is important for injectors, as placing fillers too deeply in some areas may risk nerve compression.

How Can We Restore Deep Fat Loss?

1. Dermal Fillers (Hyaluronic Acid or Biostimulatory Fillers)
Cheek Fillers: Replace volume in deep medial cheek fat to restore youthful contouring.

Tear Trough Fillers : Support the SOOF, reducing under-eye hollowing.

Chin & Jawline Fillers : Compensate for deep fat loss in the lower face.

2. Fat Grafting

Autologous fat transfer from another area of the body to restore volume in deep fat compartments. Provides a longer-lasting result but requires a surgical procedure.

3. PRP (Platelet-Rich Plasma)

Stimulates collagen and fat cell regeneration, slowing down volume loss.

Conclusion: The Deep Fat Pads as the Foundation of Facial Youth

The deep fat pads serve as the core structural support of the face, ensuring fullness and harmony between facial compartments. With aging, volume loss and downward migration of these fat pads result in hollowing, sagging, and deepened folds.

By strategically replacing lost volume in deep fat compartments using fillers or fat grafting, we can restore youthful proportions and prevent the tell-tale signs of aging.

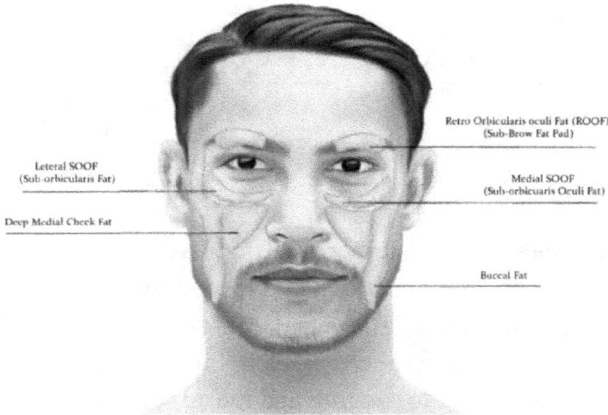

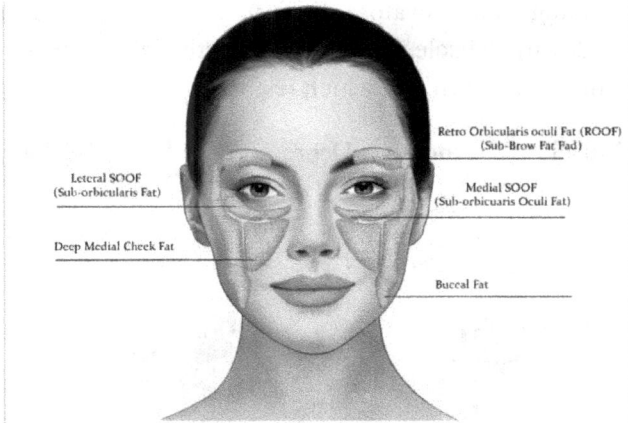

Chapter 12: Facial Muscles: The Lifting and Depressing Forces of the Face

Facial muscles are unique because they are directly attached to the skin rather than just bone. This allows them to create expressions, movement, and facial contouring. However, as we age, these muscles weaken, stretch, and undergo functional changes, contributing to sagging and the appearance of wrinkles.

Understanding the elevator (lifting) muscles and depressor (pulling down) muscles is key to aesthetic treatments like botulinum toxin and fillers, which restore balance to the face.

Facial Muscles: Elevators vs. Depressor

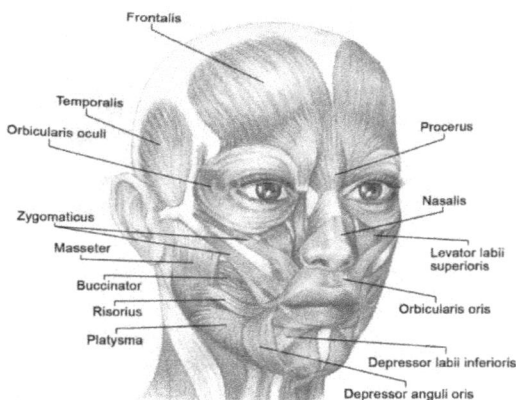

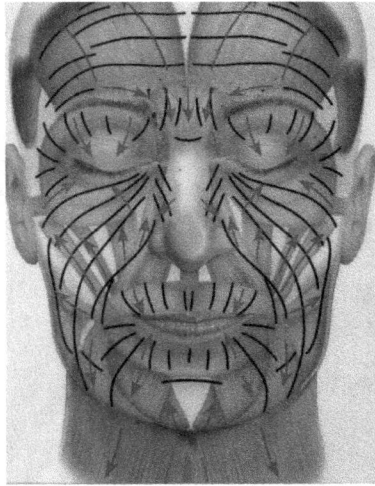

Direction of Muscle Movement: Red arrows- direction of muscle, Black Lines – wrinkles that form because of the continual movement.

Facial muscles can be divided into two main groups:

1. Elevator (Lifting) Muscles

These muscles lift the face and contribute to a youthful, open, and elevated appearance.

Frontalis : Lifts the eyebrows, creating a more alert and youthful expression.

Zygomaticus Major & Minor : Elevate the cheeks and corners of the mouth (important for smiling).

Levator Labii Superioris : Lifts the upper lip, affecting lip height and smile dynamics.

Levator Anguli Oris; Elevates the corners of the mouth (reduces marionette lines).

Orbicularis Oculi (Upper Fibers) : Helps raise the cheeks when smiling.

2. Depressor (Pulling Down) Muscles

These muscles pull the face downward, contributing to sagging, deepened folds, and an aged appearance.

Depressor Anguli Oris (DAO) : Pulls down the corners of the mouth, contributing to a sad or tired look.

Depressor Labii Inferioris : Lowers the lower lip, exposing the lower teeth when speaking or frowning.

Platysma : A thin muscle in the neck that pulls the jawline downward, contributing to jowls and neck bands.

Orbicularis Oris (Lower Fibers) : Pulls the lips downward, contributing to vertical lip lines.

Mentalis : Pulls the chin upwards and can cause chin dimpling when hyperactive.

What Happens to Facial Muscles as We Age?

1. Muscle Laxity & Weakness

Elevator muscles weaken, leading to brow drooping, cheek descent, and a downturned mouth.

The depressor muscles remain strong, pulling the face downward even more.

2. Overuse of Certain Muscles

The frontalis muscle (forehead) overworks to compensate for sagging brows, leading to horizontal forehead lines.

The orbicularis oculi (around the eyes) contracts repeatedly, causing crowfeet.

The platysma becomes more active, causing neck bands and loss of jawline definition.

3. Loss of Fat & Bone Support

When the fat pads shrink and the bone resorbs, the muscles lose their anchoring, leading to sagging.

The orbicularis oris (mouth muscle) becomes hyperactive, creating lip wrinkles.

How Does Botulinum Toxin Work on Muscles?

The Science of Botulinum Toxin: Muscle Relaxation at the Neuromuscular Junction

Botulinum toxin is a neurotoxin that temporarily blocks nerve signals to muscles, preventing them from contracting.

1. Normally, when a nerve sends a signal to a muscle, it releases acetylcholine, a neurotransmitter that triggers muscle contraction.

2. Botulinum toxin blocks the release of acetylcholine, preventing the muscle from contracting fully.

3. Over time, the muscle relaxes, smoothing out wrinkles and reducing the downward pull of depressor muscles.

Where Botulinum Toxin is Used to Balance Elevators & Depressors

Forehead Lines   Botulinum toxin weakens the frontalis, reducing horizontal forehead wrinkles.

Frown Lines (Glabella) : Relaxing the corrugator and procerus muscles prevents the dynamic lines.

Crow's Feet : Softens wrinkles around the eyes by relaxing the orbicularis oculi.

Downturned Mouth : Weakening the DAO (depressor anguli oris) helps lift the corners of the mouth.

Brow Lift : Strategic botulinum toxin placement relaxes the depressor muscles while allowing the frontalis to lift the brows.

Neck Bands : Injecting the platysma reduces banding and improves jawline definition.

Conclusion: Balancing Facial Muscles for Youthful Results

Understanding the relationship between lifting and depressing muscles is key to non-surgical facial rejuvenation. As we age, elevator muscles weaken, depressors dominate, and dynamic wrinkles form.

By strategically using botulinum toxin, we can relax overactive depressor muscles, allowing the elevators to function more effectively resulting in a natural, lifted, and youthful appearance.

Chapter 13: The Superficial Musculoaponeurotic System (SMAS) in Facial Anatomy

The Superficial Musculoaponeurotic System (SMAS) is a crucial anatomical structure in the face, playing a significant role in facial expressions and aging. Understanding its function, the effects of aging, and available treatments is essential for both medical professionals and individuals considering facial rejuvenation procedures.

What is the SMAS?

The SMAS is a fibrous network of tissue that envelops the facial muscles and connects them to the dermal layer of the skin. It extends from the neck to the forehead, providing support and facilitating coordinated facial movements. This layer is integral to transmitting the activity of facial muscles to the skin surface, enabling expressions such as smiling, frowning, and other dynamic movements.

Function of the SMAS

The primary functions of the SMAS include:

1. Structural Support: It maintains facial contour by anchoring the skin to the underlying musculature, ensuring that facial features remain in their proper positions.

2. Facial Expression: By connecting facial muscles to the skin, the SMAS allows for the transmission of muscle contractions to the skin surface, facilitating a wide range of expressions.

3. Distribution of Facial Fat: The SMAS plays a role in the distribution and compartmentalization of facial fat, contributing to the overall volume and shape of the face.

Aging and the SMAS

As the face ages, several changes occur within the SMAS:

1. **Loss of Elasticity**: The SMAS loses its elasticity and strength, diminishing its ability to support the overlying skin and soft tissues.
2. **Descent of Facial Tissues**: Due to gravity and weakened support, the SMAS and attached structures may descend, leading to sagging cheeks, jowls, and deepened nasolabial folds.
3. **Volume Loss**: Changes in the SMAS can affect the distribution of facial fat, resulting in hollowing of certain areas and contributing to an aged appearance.

These alterations contribute significantly to the visible signs of facial aging, such as sagging skin and loss of definition in the jawline and neck.

Treatment Options Involving the SMAS

Addressing age-related changes in the SMAS can be achieved through various interventions:

1. SMAS Facelift

A SMAS facelift is a surgical procedure that targets the SMAS layer to restore a youthful facial appearance. During the procedure:

Incisions are made along the hairline and around the ears.

The SMAS layer is carefully lifted, tightened, and repositioned to elevate sagging tissues and improve facial contours.

Excess skin is removed, and the remaining skin is rewrapped smoothly over the face.

This technique provides natural-looking results by addressing both deep structural support and superficial skin laxity.

2. Micro-Botulinum Toxin (Micro-Botox) Injections

Micro-Botox involves injecting diluted botulinum toxin into the superficial layers of the skin and the SMAS. This minimally invasive treatment aims to:

Improve skin texture and tone.

Reduce fine lines and wrinkles.

Decrease pore size and oil production.

Enhance overall skin tightness.

By targeting the superficial muscle fibres and glands, Micro-Botox can provide a subtle lifting effect and rejuvenate the skin's appearance without significant downtime.

Conclusion

The SMAS is a fundamental component in facial anatomy, integral to both function and aesthetics. Aging-related changes in the SMAS contribute to common signs of facial aging, but various treatments, including SMAS facelifts and Micro-Botox injections, offer effective solutions to restore a youthful appearance. Consultation with a qualified facial plastic surgeon or dermatologist can help determine the most appropriate approach based on individual needs and goals.

CHAPTER 14: SUPERFICIAL FAT PADS IN FACIAL ANATOMY

Superficial fat pads are integral components of facial anatomy, playing a crucial role in maintaining youthful contours and expressions. Understanding their location, function, and the changes they undergo with aging is essential for effective aesthetic treatments.

Location of Superficial Fat Pads

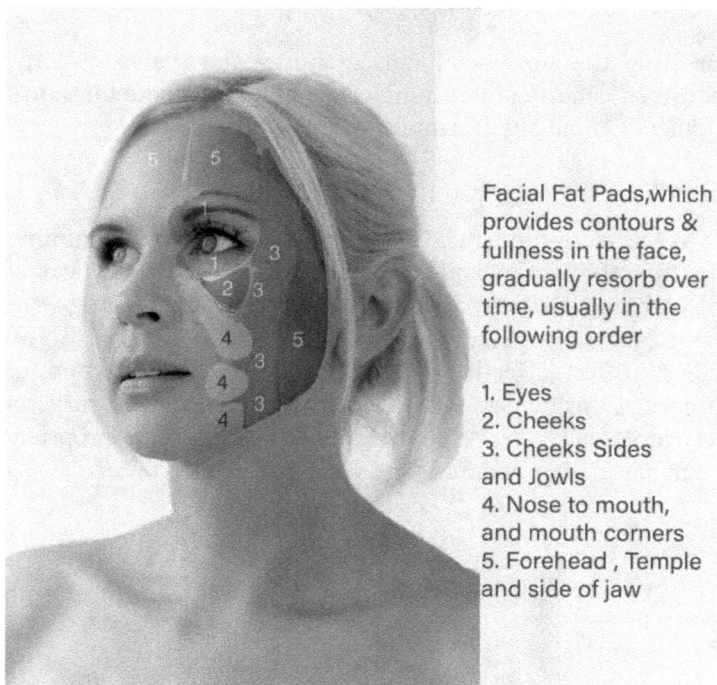

Facial Fat Pads, which provides contours & fullness in the face, gradually resorb over time, usually in the following order

1. Eyes
2. Cheeks
3. Cheeks Sides and Jowls
4. Nose to mouth, and mouth corners
5. Forehead , Temple and side of jaw

The face comprises multiple superficial fat compartments situated between the skin and the facial muscles. Key superficial fat pads include:

Infraorbital Fat Pad: Located beneath the eyes, contributing to the fullness of the lower eyelid and upper cheek.

Nasolabial Fat Pad: Positioned adjacent to the nose, extending to the corners of the mouth, influencing the prominence of the nasolabial fold.

Malar Fat Pad: Found over the cheekbones, providing midface volume and contour.

Buccal Fat Pad: Situated in the cheek area, affecting facial roundness and the definition of the cheek hollows.

Jowl Fat Pad: Located along the jawline, its descent contributes to jowl formation.

These compartments are separated by fascial septa, which help maintain the structural integrity and distribution of facial fat.

Role of Superficial Fat Pads

Superficial fat pads serve several vital functions:

1. Facial Contouring: They provide volume and shape to the face, contributing to a youthful and balanced appearance.

2. Cushioning: Acting as protective layers, they cushion underlying structures from external forces.

3. Facial Expressions: By supporting the skin and muscles, they facilitate smooth and natural facial movements.

4. Skin Support: They help maintain skin tautness by providing underlying support, preventing sagging.

Aging and Superficial Fat Pads

As we age, superficial fat pads undergo several changes:

Volume Loss: There is a reduction in fat volume, leading to hollowing in areas like the cheeks and temples.

Fat Pad Descent: Gravity and weakening connective tissues cause fat pads to shift downward, contributing to sagging and the deepening of folds such as the nasolabial crease.

Compartmental Atrophy: Selective atrophy in specific fat compartments leads to an imbalance in facial fullness, affecting overall harmony.

These changes result in common signs of facial aging, including flattened cheeks, pronounced nasolabial folds, jowling, and a general loss of youthful contours.

Treating Volume Loss in Superficial Fat Pads

Addressing volume loss involves various aesthetic interventions:

1. Dermal Fillers:

Hyaluronic Acid Fillers: Injected into specific fat compartments to restore volume, enhance contours, and smooth wrinkles.

Calcium Hydroxylapatite Fillers: Provide structural support and stimulate collagen production for longer-lasting results.

Poly-L-Lactic Acid (Sculptra): Stimulates collagen synthesis, gradually improving volume and skin texture over time.

2. Fat Grafting (Autologous Fat Transfer):

Procedure: Involves harvesting fat from another part of the body (e.g., abdomen or thighs) and injecting it into deficient facial areas.

Benefits: Utilizes the patient's tissue, reducing the risk of allergic reactions and providing natural, long-lasting results.

3. Energy-Based Devices:

Ultrasound (Ultherapy): Delivers focused ultrasound energy to stimulate deep tissue tightening and lift sagging areas.

Radiofrequency (Thermage): Uses radiofrequency energy to heat the deeper skin layers, promoting collagen remodelling and skin tightening.

4. Emerging Treatments:

Renuva: A regenerative injectable that uses donated human adipose tissue to restore the body's fat, offering a natural volumizing effect.

Facial Fat Transfer: A procedure gaining popularity for restoring facial volume, especially after significant weight loss or aging-related fat loss.

The choice of treatment depends on individual patient factors, including the extent of volume loss, skin quality, and aesthetic goals. A thorough consultation with a qualified aesthetic practitioner is essential to develop a personalized treatment plan.

Understanding the role of superficial fat pads and the impact of aging on these structures is crucial for effective facial rejuvenation. By restoring lost volume and addressing structural changes, aesthetic treatments can help maintain or recreate youthful facial contours and harmony.

Chapter 15: The Role of Facial Septa in the Formation of Facial Folds

Facial septa are integral components of facial anatomy, playing a significant role in the formation of facial folds and the overall aging process. Understanding their locations, functions, and the changes they undergo with age is essential for effective aesthetic treatments.

Locations and Functions of Facial Septa

Facial septa are fibrous partitions that compartmentalize the facial fat pads, providing structural support and maintaining the organization of facial tissues. They extend from the deeper facial structures to the skin, anchoring and separating various fat compartments. This compartmentalization allows for the independent movement of facial tissues, facilitating expressions and maintaining skin tension.

Aging and Its Impact on Facial Septa

As we age, several changes occur within the facial septa:

Loss of Elasticity: The septa lose their elasticity and strength, leading to decreased support for the overlying skin and soft tissues.

Descent of Facial Tissues: Weakened septa allow facial fat pads to shift downward, resulting in sagging and the deepening of facial folds, such as the nasolabial folds and marionette lines.

Formation of Wrinkles and Folds: The redistribution and descent of facial tissues contribute to the appearance of wrinkles and pronounced folds, altering facial contours. These structural changes are key contributors to the visible signs of facial aging.

Treatment of Facial Folds: Subcision with Cannula and Filler Augmentation

To address facial folds resulting from septal weakening and tissue descent, a combination of subcision and dermal filler augmentation can be employed:

Subcision with Cannula

Subcision is a minimally invasive surgical technique used to release fibrotic strands tethering the skin to deeper structures, thereby elevating depressed scars or folds. The procedure involves:

1. Insertion of a Blunt-Tipped Cannula: A blunt cannula is inserted beneath the skin to minimize trauma and reduce the risk of complications.

2. Release of Fibrous Attachments: The cannula is maneuvered to sever the fibrous septa responsible for the depression, allowing the skin to lift.

3. Stimulation of Collagen Production: The controlled injury promotes collagen synthesis, aiding in the long-term improvement of skin texture and elasticity.

Subcision with a blunt cannula is preferred over sharp needles due to its increased safety profile, reduced pain, and decreased risk of bruising.

Filler Augmentation

Following subcision, dermal fillers can be injected to restore volume and enhance facial contours:

Hyaluronic Acid Fillers: Commonly used to provide immediate volume restoration and hydration.

Calcium Hydroxylapatite Fillers: Offer longer-lasting results and stimulate collagen production.

The combination of subcision and filler augmentation addresses both the structural tethering and volume loss associated with facial folds, resulting in a smoother and more youthful appearance. Understanding the role of facial septa in facial anatomy is crucial for effectively treating facial folds. By employing techniques such as subcision with a cannula and filler augmentation, practitioners can achieve significant improvements in facial aesthetics, addressing both the underlying structural causes and surface manifestations of aging.

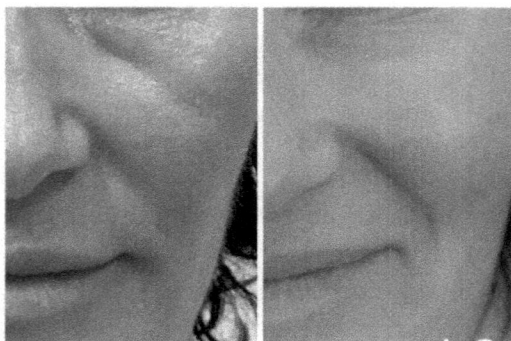

CHAPTER 16: SKIN STRUCTURE, AGING, AND REJUVENATION TREATMENTS

The skin, the body's largest organ, serves as a protective barrier and plays a crucial role in overall health. Understanding its structure, the changes it undergoes with aging, and the available treatments can help maintain its function and appearance.

Skin Structure

The skin comprises three primary layers:

1. **Epidermis**: The outermost layer, providing a barrier against environmental factors and regulating water loss.

2. **Dermis**: Located beneath the epidermis, containing collagen and elastin fibres that provide strength and elasticity.

3. **Hypodermis (Subcutaneous Layer):** The deepest layer, consisting of fat and connective tissue, offering insulation and cushioning.

Aging and Its Effects on the Skin

As we age, the skin undergoes intrinsic (natural aging) and extrinsic (environmental factors) changes:

Thinning: The epidermis and dermis become thinner, leading to increased fragility.

Loss of Elasticity: Reduction in elastin fibers causes the skin to sag and form wrinkles.

Decreased Collagen Production: Lower collagen levels result in reduced skin firmness and the development of fine lines.

Dryness: Diminished oil production leads to drier skin.

Pigmentation Changes: Age spots and uneven skin tone emerge due to prolonged sun exposure.

These changes are influenced by factors such as genetics, sun exposure, smoking, and diet.

Skin Rejuvenation Treatments

Various treatments aim to counteract the effects of aging and restore skin vitality:

1. Platelet-Rich Plasma (PRP) Therapy

PRP involves injecting concentrated platelets from the patient's blood into the skin to stimulate collagen production and cell regeneration, improving texture and tone.

2. Microneedling

This minimally invasive procedure uses fine needles to create micro-injuries in the skin, promoting collagen and elastin production. It addresses scars, wrinkles, and enlarged pores.

3. Chemical Peels

Chemical solutions are applied to exfoliate the skin's outer layers, revealing smoother, more even-toned skin beneath. They vary in strength and target issues like pigmentation and fine lines.

4. Laser Treatments

BroadBand Light (BBL): Uses light energy to target pigmentation, redness, and improve skin texture.

Laser Genesis: A non-invasive laser that heats the dermis to stimulate collagen production, reducing fine lines and promoting an even complexion.

5. LED Light Therapy

Utilizes specific light wavelengths to penetrate the skin, reducing inflammation and promoting healing. It's effective for acne, redness, and signs of aging.

6. Cosmeceuticals

Topical products containing active ingredients like retinoids, peptides, exosomes and antioxidants aim to improve skin health and appearance.

7. Skin Boosters

Injectable treatments that deliver hyaluronic acid and other nutrients to hydrate and improve skin quality, resulting in a plumper and more radiant appearance.

8. Mesotherapy

Involves microinjections of vitamins, enzymes, and plant extracts to rejuvenate and tighten skin.

Such as NCTF 135: A mesotherapy solution containing hyaluronic acid, vitamins, amino acids, and antioxidants. It revitalizes and hydrates the skin, improving elasticity and radiance.

9. Glass Skin Trend

Originating from Korea, this trend focuses on achieving exceptionally smooth, clear, and luminous skin through a combination of skincare routines and treatments emphasizing hydration and layering of products.

Achieving the coveted glass skin's appearance by exceptionally smooth, clear, and luminous skin has led to the development of innovative injectable treatments designed to enhance skin hydration, texture, and overall radiance. These treatments work beneath the skin surface to promote a youthful, dewy complexion.

A. Skin Boosters:

As mentioned before .Skin boosters are injectable treatments that deliver hyaluronic acid (HA) and other nourishing substances directly into the skin's middle layer (mesoderm). Unlike traditional dermal fillers that add volume, skin boosters focus on improving skin quality by enhancing hydration and elasticity.

Procedure: A series of microinjections administers a stabilized HA formulation into the skin, promoting deep hydration and stimulating collagen production.

Benefits: Improved skin texture, increased elasticity, and a radiant glow.

Duration: Results typically last up to six months, with maintenance sessions recommended biannually.

B. Skin Botox (Mesobotox)

Originating in South Korea, skin Botox involves microinjections of diluted botulinum toxin (Botox) into the superficial layers of the skin, rather than deeper facial muscles. This technique aims to refine skin texture and minimize pore appearance without affecting facial expressions.

Procedure: A fine needle delivers small amounts of diluted Botox just beneath the skin's surface.

Benefits: Reduction in fine lines, decreased oil production, minimized pore size, and a smoother, glass-like skin appearance.

Duration: Effects typically last three to four months, with treatments repeated as needed.

It's important to note that while skin Botox can provide a temporary glass skin effect, it requires maintenance treatments to sustain the results

C. Rejuran (Salmon DNA) Therapy:

Rejuran is an injectable treatment containing polynucleotides derived from salmon DNA, known for their regenerative properties. This therapy aims to repair damaged skin, improve elasticity, and provide deep hydration.

Procedure: Microinjections deliver the polynucleotide-rich solution into the dermis.

Benefits: Enhanced skin repair, increased elasticity, improved hydration, and a youthful glow.

Duration: A series of treatments is often recommended, with effects lasting up to six months post-treatment.

Rejuran has gained popularity in Asia and is now making its way into Western skincare routines, offering benefits for addressing issues such as dryness, fine lines, and uneven skin tone.

Considerations:

Consultation: It's essential to consult with a qualified medical professional to determine the most appropriate treatment based on individual skin concerns and goals.

Side Effects: Potential side effects may include temporary redness, swelling, or bruising at the injection sites.

Maintenance: Regular maintenance sessions are often required to sustain the desired glass skin effect.

These injectable treatments offer promising results for those seeking to achieve a glass-like skin appearance, providing deep hydration and enhancing overall skin quality.

CHAPTER 17: WRINKLES, LINES AND LAUGHS

Let's face it-lines happen. We smile, we squint, we sleep (hopefully), and our faces keep score. But not all lines are created equal. In this chapter, we'll decode the different types of wrinkles, what causes them, and what can be done-clinically and cleverly-to soften or even erase their presence.

Dynamic Lines: The Lines of Expression These are the first ones to show up, often while you're still young and animated. They're called dynamic because they appear with movement-when you frown, laugh, or raise your brows.

Forehead lines: Those horizontal "surprise!" lines from raising your eyebrows.- Glabellar lines (the '11s'): Between the brows-thanks, frowning.- Crow's feet: The fan of fine lines at the outer corners of the eyes from smiling or squinting.

Treatment: These respond beautifully to wrinkle relaxers like Botox, Dysport, or Xeomin. By calming the muscles, you soften the lines-and yes, you can still express yourself (just minus the furrows).

Static Lines: When They Stick Around Over time, dynamic lines become static-meaning they're visible even when your face is resting. But wait, there's more: We also develop sleep lines, those vertical creases that have nothing to do with emotion and everything to do with how you face-plant your pillow.

Sleep Lines: The Quiet Saboteurs- Common spots: Between the brows, across the top lip, along the cheeks, and the dreaded marionette lines.- They often appear worse on one side-yes, the side you sleep on.- Tip: If you're married, it's usually the side facing away from your husband (insert dramatic sigh here).

These lines don't respond well to wrinkle relaxers, because they're not caused by movement-they're etched into your skin like creases in satin from years of being smooshed into a pillow.

Line Work: Filling in the Story When relaxers can't help, dermal fillers step in. But not just any filler-you need one that's soft, flexible, and designed for fine superficial lines.

Top Products for Line Work:

Teosyal RHA 1: A standout for treating fine lines thanks to its high stretch and low viscosity. Great around the lips and eyes.

Belotero Balance: Excellent for feathering into superficial lines without Tyndall effect.

Restylane Fynesse or Vital Light: Especially helpful for crepey areas with fine etched lines.

Juvéderm Volbella (used lightly): Can work under the eyes or lips with caution.

NCTF 135 HA (for skin quality): Not a filler per se, but supports hydration and fine line softening.

The Fern Technique:

One of the most refined approaches to line work is the fern technique, developed to mimic the natural direction of collagen and elastin fibers in the dermis.

The injector creates tiny, branching lines of filler-like fern leaves-along the wrinkle's path.

This technique disperses the filler in a way that supports the skin without creating bulk.

It works especially well for smokers' lines, accordion lines, and sleep creases, particularly around the top lip, chin, and cheeks.

It's delicate work-think calligraphy for the face-and best done with soft fillers like RHA 1 or Belotero Soft. It requires finesse, and not all injectors are trained in this technique, so always seek out someone experienced.

Takeaway Tips:

Relaxers work best for movement lines-get in early before they etch in.

Fillers are for lines that don't move but refuse to leave.

Soft, stretchy fillers and techniques like the fern method offer natural results when done right.

And yes-how you sleep matters. A silk pillowcase helps, but maybe don't roll away from your spouse every single night.

Sleep Smart, Not Scrunched

Want to reduce those pesky sleep lines? Try this:

Place a pillow under your knees and a travel pillow under your neck—you'll feel like you're in a side-sleeping, fetal position, but you're actually on your back. This position is surprisingly comfortable and reduces pressure on your face.

If you must sleep on your side, use a C-shaped travel pillow and rest your face in the open space. Your cheek stays free-floating—not squished—helping prevent those deep creases from forming overnight.

CHAPTER 18: THE NECK ANATOMY, AGING, AND REJUVENATION TREATMENTS

The neck, a vital yet often overlooked region, exhibits unique anatomical features and aging patterns distinct from the face. Understanding its layered structure and the available treatments can aid in maintaining its youthful appearance.

Anatomy of the Neck

The neck's anatomy comprises several layers, each contributing to its function and aesthetics:

1. Skin: The outermost layer, providing a protective barrier.

2. Superficial Cervical Fascia: Located just beneath the skin, this layer contains:

Neurovascular structures supplying the skin

Superficial veins, such as the external jugular vein

Superficial lymph nodes

Fat

The platysma muscle

3. Platysma Muscle: A broad, superficial muscle extending from the chest and shoulder region upward to the lower face, playing a role in facial expressions and contributing to the neck's contour.

4. Deep Cervical Fascia: Situated beneath the superficial fascia and platysma, this fascia is organized into several layers:

Investing Layer: Encircles the entire neck, enclosing the trapezius and sternocleidomastoid muscles.

Pretracheal Layer: Surrounds the trachea, esophagus, and thyroid gland.

Prevertebral Layer: Envelops the vertebral column and associated deep muscles.

These fascial layers compartmentalize neck structures, providing support and facilitating movement.

In comparison, the face features the superficial musculoaponeurotic system (SMAS), a continuous fibromuscular layer that differs from the neck's fascial composition.

Aging of the Neck

The neck undergoes specific changes as part of the aging process:

Skin Laxity: Decreased collagen and elastin production lead to looser, sagging skin.

Muscle Banding: The platysma muscle may become more prominent, forming vertical bands.

Fat Accumulation or Loss: Uneven fat distribution can result in a double chin or a gaunt appearance.

Sun Damage: Chronic exposure contributes to wrinkles, pigmentation changes, and a leathery texture.

These changes can cause the neck to age differently from the face, often becoming a noticeable indicator of aging.

Rejuvenation Treatments for the Neck

Various treatments aim to address the signs of neck aging, focusing on skin tightening, volume restoration, and texture improvement:

1. Platelet-Rich Plasma (PRP) Therapy

PRP involves injecting concentrated platelets from the patient's blood into the neck skin to stimulate collagen production and enhance skin quality.

Benefits: Improved skin texture, increased elasticity, and a more youthful appearance.

Procedure: Blood is drawn, processed to concentrate platelets, and then injected into targeted areas.

Considerations: Multiple sessions may be required for optimal results.

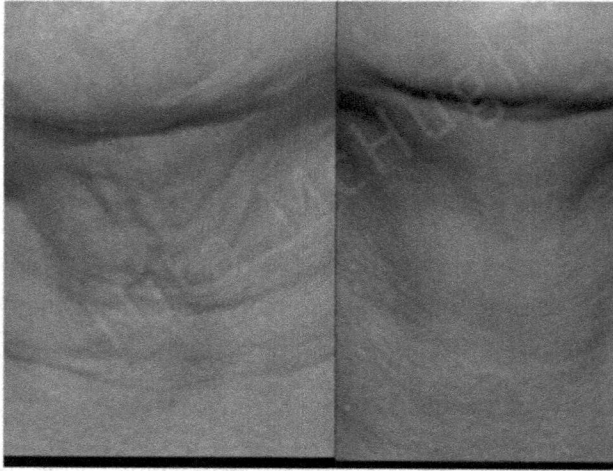

Neck after 3 sessions of PRP

2. Hyperdiluted Sculptra (Poly-L-Lactic Acid)

Sculptra is a biostimulatory filler that, when hyperdiluted, can be used to treat larger surface areas like the neck.

Benefits: Stimulates collagen production, leading to gradual skin tightening and improved texture.

Procedure: The diluted solution is injected into the dermis, promoting collagen synthesis over time.

Considerations: Results develop gradually over several months, with effects lasting up to two years.

3. Hyperdiluted Radiesse (Calcium Hydroxylapatite)

Radiesse, another biostimulatory filler, can be diluted for use in the neck area.

Benefits: Provides immediate volume and stimulates collagen production for long-term improvement.

Procedure: The hyperdiluted filler is injected to cover larger areas, enhancing skin texture and firmness.

Considerations: Typically requires multiple treatments spaced weeks apart.

4. Skin Boosters

Injectable treatments that deliver hyaluronic acid and other nutrients to the skin.

Benefits: Deep hydration, improved skin elasticity, and a radiant appearance.

Procedure: Microinjections are administered into the superficial dermis.

Considerations: Maintenance treatments are often needed to sustain results.

5. Profhilo

A unique injectable hyaluronic acid treatment designed to improve skin laxity.

Benefits: Enhances skin hydration and stimulates collagen and elastin production, resulting in firmer skin.

Procedure: Injected into specific points, allowing the product to diffuse and rejuvenate the skin.

Considerations: Typically involves two sessions spaced a month apart, with effects lasting up to six months.

6. Fine Line Fillers

Utilizing very fine fillers designed to integrate smoothly into the tissue.

Benefits: Targets horizontal lines and creases without creating lumps, resulting in a natural look.

Procedure: Injected superficially to smooth out lines and creases.

Submental Fat (Double Chin)

Submental fat, commonly known as a "double chin," can be caused by various factors, including:

Causes of Submental Fat

1. **Genetics** – Some people are predisposed to storing fat under the chin.

2. **Aging** – Loss of skin elasticity and fat redistribution can contribute.

3. **Weight Gain** – Excess fat deposits accumulate in various areas, including the submental region.

4. **Posture** – Poor posture can weaken neck muscles, making fat more noticeable.

5. **Hormonal Changes** – Hormones and metabolism shifts can impact fat storage.

Treatment Options for Reducing Submental Fat

1. Belkyra (Kybella in the USA)

• Active ingredient: Deoxycholic Acid (DCA)

• Works by breaking down fat cells, which are then absorbed by the body.

- Sessions Required: Usually 3 to 4 sessions (4-6 weeks apart)

- Downtime: Swelling is common for 1-2 weeks, with tenderness and firmness in the treated area.

- Best For: Small-to-moderate fat pockets.

2. Compounded PPC + Deoxycholic Acid (Mesotherapy)

- Similar to Belkyra/Kybella but may have a different formulation.

- Main ingredients: Phosphatidylcholine (PPC) + Deoxycholic Acid (DCA).

- Swelling/Downtime: Similar to Belkyra, with noticeable swelling lasting 5-14 days.

- Sessions Required: Typically 3+ sessions.

3. CoolSculpting (Cryolipolysis)

- Freezes fat cells, which are naturally eliminated over time.

- Non-invasive, minimal downtime but may take 8-12 weeks for full results.

- Sessions Required: Usually 2+ sessions.

- Best For: Mild-to-moderate fat deposits.

4. Liposculpture (Liposuction for Chin)

- Surgical option to suction out excess fat.

- Downtime: Bruising and swelling for 1-2 weeks.

- Best For: Significant fat deposits or those seeking immediate, permanent results.

5. FaceTite (Radiofrequency-Assisted Liposuction)

- Uses RF energy to melt fat and tighten skin simultaneously.

- Minimally invasive with 1-2 weeks of downtime.

- Best For: Fat reduction with skin laxity improvement.

6. PRP for Small Fat Deposits & Skin Tightening

- Platelet-Rich Plasma (PRP) can tighten skin and improve collagen around the jawline.

- Works best for mild cases or in combination with other treatments.

- Sessions Required: Usually 3+ sessions.

Choosing the Right Treatment

- For minimal fat + skin laxity: PRP or FaceTite.

- For moderate fat: Belkyra/Kybella, PPC/Deoxycholic, or CoolSculpting.

- For large fat deposits: Liposuction or FaceTite.

- For immediate results: Liposculpture or FaceTite.

- For gradual, non-invasive reduction: CoolSculpting or Belkyra.

Tech Neck

Tech neck lines are horizontal wrinkles on the neck caused by constantly looking down at screens, leading to collagen breakdown and premature aging. Factors such as poor posture, skin dehydration, and repetitive movement contribute to their formation.

Since the neck has thinner skin and fewer oil glands, it is more prone to wrinkles and laxity.

While aging plays a role, lifestyle habits accelerate the process. Addressing these lines requires a combination of treatments that hydrate, tighten, and stimulate collagen production to restore skin smoothness and elasticity.

A powerful approach to treating tech neck lines is combining PRP (Platelet-Rich Plasma) and Skin Boosters. PRP stimulates collagen production and strengthens skin over time, while skin boosters provide deep hydration, smoothing static wrinkles.

Together, they enhance skin elasticity, hydration, and overall texture.

A recommended treatment plan involves three sessions spaced over a few months, with visible improvements in hydration within weeks and long-term collagen repair over several months.

Alongside treatment, good posture, sun protection, retinol, and hydration play key roles in prevention.

With the right combination of treatments and lifestyle changes, tech neck lines can be significantly reduced, leaving the neck looking youthful and rejuvenated.

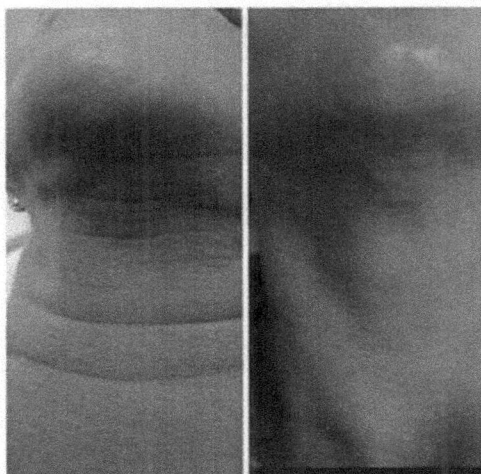

CHAPTER 19: THE HAND REJUVENATION

Aging hands often reveal a person's age just as much if not more than the face. Over time, the skin on the hands becomes thinner, veins and tendons become more prominent, and volume loss creates a bony appearance. The natural aging process, combined with sun exposure and environmental factors, leads to a loss of collagen, elasticity, and hydration, making the hands look fragile and wrinkled.

Fortunately, advancements in aesthetic medicine offer several effective treatments to rejuvenate aging hands, restoring volume, improving skin quality, and enhancing overall appearance.

2 treatments of Radiesse with cannula

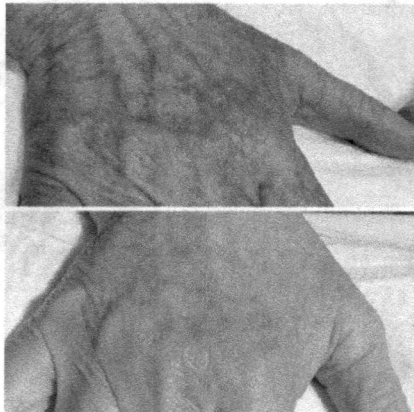

Platelet-Rich Plasma (PRP) therapy is a natural approach to hand rejuvenation. By using the patient's own blood, PRP harnesses growth factors to stimulate collagen production, improve skin texture, and enhance hydration. The regenerative properties of PRP can reduce crepiness and improve overall skin resilience, making it a great option for those seeking a natural, gradual improvement.

Dermal Fillers: Restoring Volume

Injectable fillers provide an immediate solution to volume loss in the hands. By replenishing lost fullness, fillers help smooth the skeletal appearance, reducing the visibility of veins and tendons. Hyaluronic acid fillers, calcium hydroxylapatite (Radiesse), and poly-L-lactic acid (Sculptra) are commonly used for this purpose. Each has unique benefits:

Hyaluronic Acid Fillers: Provide instant hydration and volume, though results may be temporary.

Sculptra: Works gradually by stimulating collagen production, creating a more natural, long-term improvement.

Radiesse: My personal favourite for hand rejuvenation. Unlike other fillers, Radiesse not only stimulates collagen but also has an opaque quality, making it excellent for disguising prominent veins and tendons. It offers both immediate and long-term benefits, giving hands a smoother, more youthful appearance.

Skin Boosters: Hydration and Glow

For those with crepey, thin skin, skin boosters such as polynucleotides or micro-injections of hyaluronic acid can deeply hydrate the skin, improving elasticity and texture. These treatments work well in combination with fillers to enhance overall hand rejuvenation.

Choosing the Right Treatment

The best approach to hand rejuvenation often involves a combination of treatments tailored to the individual's needs. While PRP and skin boosters improve skin quality over time, fillers like Radiesse provide immediate structural support and collagen stimulation. Protecting the hands with sunscreen, moisturizers, and a good skincare routine further enhances the results.

Aging hands no longer have to be a telltale sign of age. With the right combination of treatments, hands can remain as youthful and elegant as the rest of you.

CHAPTER 20: THE DÉCOLLETAGE

The décolletage , encompassing the upper chest area between the neck and the breasts, is often exposed yet frequently neglected in skincare routines. Understanding its anatomy, the effects of aging, and preventive measures can help maintain its youthful appearance.

Anatomy of the Décolletage

The skin of the décolletage is notably thin and delicate, with fewer oil glands and less subcutaneous fat compared to other body areas. This makes it more susceptible to environmental damage and the early onset of wrinkles. The underlying structures include the pectoral muscles and connective tissues that provide support to the skin and breast tissue.

Aging of the Décolletage

As we age, the décolletage undergoes several changes:

Loss of Elasticity: Decreased collagen and elastin production lead to skin laxity and the formation of wrinkles.

Hyperpigmentation: Prolonged sun exposure can cause age spots and uneven skin tone.

Volume Loss: Reduction in subcutaneous fat can result in a less plump appearance.

Wrinkling from Sleep Positions: Sleeping on one's side can cause the breasts to press together, leading to vertical creases in the décolletage area.

Preventive Measures for Side Sleepers

For individuals who prefer side sleeping, the following strategies can help prevent sleep-induced chest wrinkles:

Breast Support Pillows: Specialized pillows, such as the Intimia Breast Pillow, are designed to be worn between the breasts during sleep. They help maintain breast separation, reducing skin creasing and discomfort.

Supportive Sleepwear: Wearing a supportive bra or specially designed sleepwear can minimize breast movement and skin folding during sleep.

Rejuvenation Treatments for the Décolletage.

Various treatments can address signs of aging in the décolletage:

 Topical Retinoids: Applying retinoid creams can stimulate collagen production, improving skin texture and reducing fine lines.

Chemical Peels: Controlled application of chemical solutions exfoliates the skin, promoting the growth of new, smoother skin and reducing pigmentation issues.

Laser Resurfacing: Laser treatments can resurface the skin, remove discoloration, smooth lines, and tighten loose skin.

Micro needling : This procedure creates micro-injuries in the skin, stimulating collagen production and improving skin texture.

Injectable Fillers: Hyaluronic acid-based fillers, can effectively reduce the appearance of lines and wrinkles on the chest.

Sculptra (Poly-L-Lactic Acid): Sculptra injections stimulate collagen production, improving wrinkles and crepey skin in the décolletage area with natural, long-lasting results.

Silicone Patches: Medical-grade silicone patches can be applied to the décolletage to hydrate the skin and reduce the appearance of wrinkles. Products like Wrinkles Schminkles have gained popularity for their effectiveness in smoothing chest wrinkles.

Incorporating these preventive measures and treatments can help maintain the youthful appearance of the décolletage .

CHAPTER 21: THE STRUCTURE OF LIPS, AGING EFFECTS, AND REJUVENATION TREATMENTS

The lips are a central feature of facial aesthetics, playing a significant role in expressions and overall appearance. Understanding their anatomy, the aging process, and available treatments can aid in maintaining or restoring their youthful allure.

Anatomy of the Lips

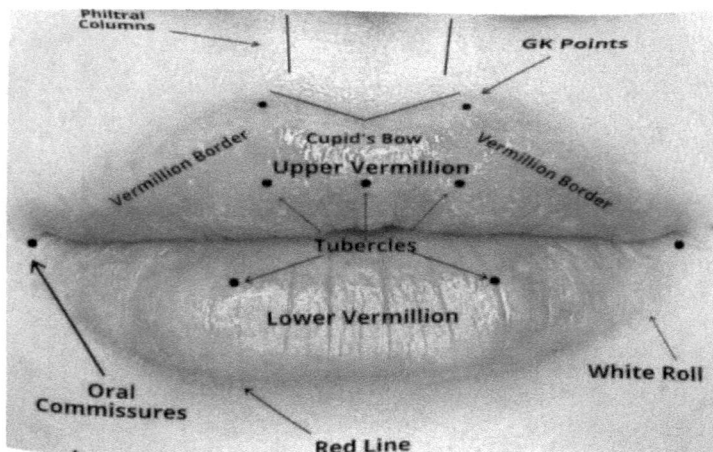

The lips are composed of several distinct anatomical components:

Vermilion Zone: The pigmented area of the lips, lacking sweat and sebaceous glands, making it prone to dryness.

Vermilion Border: The demarcation line between the vermilion zone and the surrounding skin, often highlighted by a subtle ridge known as the white roll.

Cupids Bow: The double-curve of the upper lip, contributing to its characteristic shape.

Philtrum: The vertical groove between the base of the nose and the upper lip.

Orbicularis Oris Muscle: A circular muscle encircling the mouth, essential for lip movement and function.

These structures work in harmony to facilitate speech, expression, and ingestion.

Aging of the Lips

As individuals age, the lips undergo several changes:

Volume Loss: A decrease in collagen and elastin leads to thinner lips and diminished fullness.

Lengthening of the Upper Lip: The upper lip tends to elongate over time, contributing to a flatter appearance.

Development of Fine Lines: Vertical lines, often referred to as lipstick lines • or smoker's lines • emerge due to repetitive movements and skin thinning.

Loss of Definition: The vermilion border and Cupid's bow become less distinct, reducing lip contour clarity

These alterations can result in a less youthful and vibrant appearance.

Rejuvenation Treatments

To counteract the effects of aging on the lips, several treatments are available:

1. Platelet-Rich Plasma (PRP) Therapy

PRP involves injecting concentrated platelets from the patient blood into the lips to stimulate collagen production and tissue regeneration.

Benefits: Enhances lip texture, reduces fine lines, and promotes natural fullness.

Procedure: Blood is drawn, processed to isolate platelets, and then injected into the lips.

Considerations: Results develop gradually over several weeks, with minimal risk of allergic reactions since the patient's own blood is used.

2. Dermal Fillers

Hyaluronic acid-based fillers are commonly used to restore volume and define lip contours.

Benefits: Immediate enhancement of lip fullness and shape, with the ability to target specific areas for balanced results.

Procedure: Fillers are injected into designated lip regions to achieve the desired augmentation.

Considerations: Results are temporary, typically lasting 6 to 12 months, and treatments can be adjusted to achieve subtle or more pronounced enhancements.

Consultation with a qualified medical professional is essential to determine the most appropriate treatment plan based on individual goals and anatomical considerations.

By understanding the structural changes that occur in the lips with aging and the available rejuvenation options, individuals can make informed decisions to maintain or restore a youthful and natural lip appearance.

CHAPTER 22: EARS, EYES, AND NOSE: AGING CHANGES AND REJUVENATION TREATMENTS

As we age, our ears, eyes, and nose undergo various structural and functional changes. Understanding these alterations and the available treatments can help maintain a youthful appearance and optimal function.

Aging of the Ears

Changes Observed:

Elongation and Sagging: Over time, the skin and cartilage of the ears lose elasticity, leading to elongation and sagging, particularly in the earlobes.

Wrinkling: The reduction in collagen and elastin contributes to the formation of wrinkles on the earlobes.

Treatment Options:

Dermal Fillers: Injecting hyaluronic acid-based fillers can restore volume and reduce the appearance of wrinkles in the earlobes.

Platelet-Rich Plasma (PRP) Therapy: PRP injections stimulate collagen production, enhancing skin texture and firmness in the earlobes.

Earlobe Lift Surgery: For more pronounced sagging, surgical procedures can reshape and reduce the size of the earlobes.

Aging of the Eyes

Changes Observed:

Periorbital Wrinkles: Commonly known as crow's feet, these fine lines develop around the eyes due to repetitive facial expressions and thinning skin.

Dark Circles and Hollows: Volume loss and decreased skin thickness can lead to a sunken appearance and darkening under the eyes.

Puffiness: Fluid retention and weakening of the tissues around the eyes can cause puffiness.

Eye Bags from Fluid Retention: Can Hyalase Help?

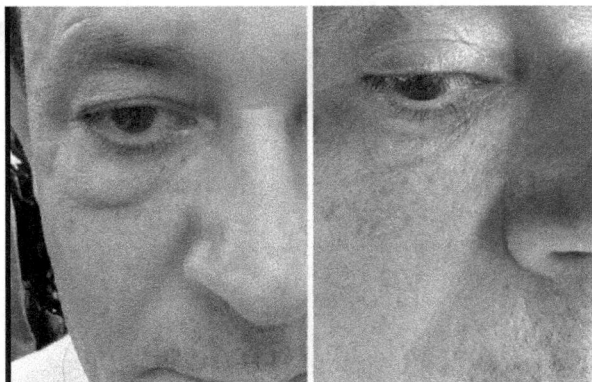

25 iu of hyalase drained the fluid build up
(no filler present).

Some under-eye puffiness is caused not by fat pads but by fluid retention due to poor lymphatic drainage. This can worsen with hay fever and allergies, as inflammation can affect drainage channels around the eyes—possibly linked to valve-like structures in the lymphatic vessels.

While true fat pads or permanent eye bags typically require lower blepharoplasty surgery for correction, fluid-based puffiness may respond to Hyalase (hyaluronidase). This enzyme can help dissolve any lingering HA filler or excess glycosaminoglycans that may be obstructing lymphatic flow, improving drainage.

Worth a trial: If there is a history of prior filler or persistent puffiness that fluctuates, a conservative dose of Hyalase may reduce swelling by improving drainage—even if no obvious filler is present.

Treatment Options:

Platelet-Rich Plasma (PRP) Therapy: PRP injections under the eyes can improve skin texture, reduce dark circles, and promote a more youthful appearance.

Laser Resurfacing: Fractional CO_2 and erbium lasers can reduce fine lines and wrinkles by promoting collagen production and resurfacing the skin.

Dermal Fillers: Hyaluronic acid-based fillers can restore volume to under-eye hollows, reducing the appearance of dark circles and providing a rejuvenated look.

Upper blepharoplasty , surgically removing excess sagging skin, and lower blepharoplasty surgically addressing fat pads that cause bags and removing excess skin .

Lifestyle Modifications: Wearing sunglasses to protect against UV rays, reducing consumption of ultra-processed foods, managing allergies, and applying retinol eye cream can help maintain youthful-looking eyes.

Aging of the Nose

Changes Observed:

Drooping Tip: The nasal tip may droop due to weakening of the supporting cartilage, leading to a lengthened appearance.

Prominent Nasolabial Folds: Volume loss around the nose can deepen the folds between the nose and mouth.

Treatment Options:

Dermal Fillers: Injecting fillers into areas like the pyriform fossa can provide support, lift the nasal tip, and soften nasolabial folds.

Rhinoplasty: Surgical intervention can correct structural changes in the nose, addressing both aesthetic and functional concerns.

Consulting with qualified medical professionals is essential to determine the most appropriate treatment plan based on individual needs and anatomical considerations

CHAPTER 23: FOREHEAD STRUCTURE, AGING, AND REJUVENATION STRATEGIES

The forehead plays a pivotal role in facial aesthetics and expressions. As we age, structural changes in the forehead can lead to concerns such as eyebrow drooping (brow ptosis) and the formation of wrinkles. Understanding the anatomy of the forehead, the aging process, and available rejuvenation treatments can aid in maintaining a youthful and refreshed appearance.

Anatomy of the Forehead

The forehead comprises several key components:

Skin: The outermost layer, providing protection and housing sensory receptors.

Subcutaneous Fat: A thin layer of fat beneath the skin that offers minimal cushioning.

Frontalis Muscle: A broad, flat muscle responsible for elevating the eyebrows and creating horizontal forehead lines during contraction.

Galea Aponeurotica: A tough, fibrous tissue layer connecting the frontalis muscle to the occipitalis muscle at the back of the head.

Periosteum: A dense layer of connective tissue covering the frontal bone, providing attachment points for muscles and ligaments.

Aging of the Forehead

With advancing age, the forehead undergoes several notable changes:

Skin Laxity: Decreased collagen and elastin production lead to reduced skin elasticity, resulting in sagging.

Volume Loss: Diminished subcutaneous fat and bone resorption contribute to a hollowed or sunken appearance.

Muscle Weakness: Over time, the frontalis muscle may weaken, exacerbating sagging and the descent of the eyebrows.

Wrinkle Formation: Repetitive muscle contractions and skin laxity cause the development of horizontal forehead lines and vertical glabellar lines (frown lines).

Eyebrow Droop (Brow Ptosis)

Brow ptosis refers to the downward displacement of the eyebrows, often resulting in a tired or stern appearance. This condition is primarily due to:

Soft Tissue Descent: Age-related weakening and stretching of the soft tissues lead to the downward movement of the brow.

Frontalis Muscle Weakness: Reduced muscle tone diminishes the ability to elevate the eyebrows effectively.

Bone Resorption: Loss of bone mass in the frontal bone can contribute to the descent of the forehead and brow structures.

The lateral (outer) portion of the eyebrow often exhibits ptosis earlier than the medial (inner) portion, contributing to a fatigued appearance.

Rejuvenation Treatments

To address the signs of aging in the forehead and brow region, several treatment options are available:

1. Sculptra® (Poly-L-Lactic Acid) Injections

Sculptra is a biostimulatory injectable that stimulates the body's natural collagen production, restoring volume and improving skin texture.

Application: While Sculptra is commonly used in areas such as the temples, cheeks, and chin, its use in the forehead is less typical due to anatomical considerations.

Benefits: When appropriately applied, Sculptra can address volume loss and enhance skin elasticity, contributing to a more youthful forehead contour.

Considerations: Treatment effects develop gradually over several months, with results lasting up to two years.

2. Hyaluronic Acid Fillers

Dermal fillers with specific rheological properties can be used to smooth forehead wrinkles and restore volume.

Application: Fillers are injected into targeted areas to fill in deep lines and compensate for volume loss.

Benefits: Immediate improvement in the appearance of wrinkles and enhanced skin hydration.

Considerations: Choosing fillers with appropriate viscosity ensures even distribution and minimizes the risk of lumpiness.

3. Neuromodulators (e.g., Botulinum Toxin)

Injectables like botulinum toxin temporarily relax the frontalis muscle, reducing the appearance of dynamic wrinkles.

Application: Administered into specific points of the forehead to diminish muscle activity.

Benefits: Effective in smoothing horizontal forehead lines and preventing the formation of deeper wrinkles.

Considerations: Overuse can lead to brow ptosis; thus, treatments should be performed by experienced practitioners.

4. Brow Lift Surgery

For more pronounced brow ptosis, surgical intervention may be considered.

Procedure: Involves repositioning the brow to a more elevated position, addressing both functional and aesthetic concerns.

Benefits: Provides long-lasting results and can significantly rejuvenate the upper face.

Considerations: Surgical risks and recovery time should be discussed with a qualified surgeon.

CHAPTER 24: THE CHIN'S ANATOMY, AGING, AND REJUVENATION STRATEGIES

The chin significantly influences facial harmony and aesthetics. As we age, the chin undergoes various structural changes affecting its appearance and function. Understanding these changes and the available treatments can help maintain or restore a youthful chin contour.

Anatomy of the Chin

The chin, or mental region, comprises several key components:

Bone: The mandible (lower jawbone) forms the bony foundation of the chin.

Muscles: The primary muscle in this area is the mentalis, which elevates and protrudes the lower lip and wrinkles the chin skin.

Skin and Subcutaneous Tissue: Overlying the muscle, the skin and connective tissues contribute to the chin's external appearance.

Aging of the Chin

With aging, the chin experiences several notable changes:

Bone Resorption: The mandible undergoes resorption, leading to a reduction in chin projection and a less defined jawline.

Muscle Activity: Overactivity of the mentalis muscle can cause chin dimpling, often referred to as an "orange peel" appearance.

Soft Tissue Changes: Loss of subcutaneous fat and skin elasticity contributes to sagging and the formation of marionette lines (melomental folds) extending from the mouth corners to the chin.

Rejuvenation Treatments

To address these aging-related changes, several treatment options are available:

1. Botulinum Toxin Injections

Injecting botulinum toxin into the mentalis muscle can relax overactivity, reducing chin dimpling and creating a smoother appearance.

Procedure: A small amount of botulinum toxin is injected directly into the mentalis muscle.

Benefits: Improves the Orange peel texture and softens the mental crease.

Considerations: Effects are temporary, typically lasting 3 to 4 months, requiring repeat treatments for maintenance.

2. Dermal Fillers

Dermal fillers can restore lost volume, enhance chin projection, and smooth marionette lines.

Procedure: Fillers are injected into specific areas of the chin and surrounding regions to add volume and structure.

Benefits: Immediate improvement in chin contour and reduction of wrinkles.

Considerations: Choosing fillers with appropriate rheological properties ensures a natural look and minimizes lumpiness.

3. Calcium Hydroxylapatite (Radiesse)

Radiesse is a filler that provides immediate volume and stimulates collagen production, making it suitable for enhancing chin structure and addressing bone loss.

Procedure: Injected into deeper layers of the chin to provide structural support.

Benefits: Restores volume, improves skin texture, and offers longer-lasting results compared to some other fillers.

Considerations: Results can last up to a year or more; some patients may experience temporary swelling or bruising.

4. Subcision with Cannula ("Happy Lift")

Marionette lines can be treated using a subcision technique with a cannula, sometimes referred to as the "Happy Lift"

Procedure: A blunt-tipped cannula is inserted under the skin to release fibrous bands causing the marionette lines, followed by filler injection to maintain the lifted appearance.

Benefits: Reduces the depth of marionette lines and restores a smoother transition between the mouth corners and chin.

Considerations: The term "happy lift" is associated with thread lifting techniques; however, in this context, it refers to the subcision method using a cannula.

5. Lip Support and Projection

As the chin bone recedes with age, the lower lip may turn inward, leading to a thinner appearance.

Procedure: Injecting fillers into the upper part of the chin can provide support and outward projection to the lower lip.

Benefits: Enhances lip fullness and restores a balanced profile.

Considerations: Careful assessment is required to achieve natural-looking results without overcorrection.

Consultation with a qualified medical professional is essential to determine the most appropriate treatment plan based on individual anatomy and aesthetic goals. Combining multiple treatments may yield optimal results in restoring a youthful chin appearance..

CHAPTER 25: EYEBROWS: AGING CHANGES AND REJUVENATION STRATEGIES

Eyebrows play a crucial role in facial expression, symmetry, and aesthetics. As we age, various changes occur in the eyebrows that can affect overall facial appearance. Understanding these changes and exploring effective rejuvenation strategies can help maintain a youthful and balanced look.

Aging and the Eyebrows

Several factors contribute to the aging of eyebrows:

Thinning and Hair Loss: Over time, eyebrows may become sparser due to hormonal changes and the natural aging process. This can result in a less defined brow, impacting facial expression.

Greying: Just like scalp hair, eyebrow hairs can lose pigment, leading to greying. This change can make the brows appear less prominent.

Drooping: The lateral (outer) portion of the eyebrow tends to sag with age due to the lack of muscle support in that area, contributing to a tired or stern appearance.

Over-Plucking: Trends from past decades, such as the thin brows popular in the 1970s, have led to over-plucking. This can result in permanent thinning, making the brows appear outdated and contributing to an aged look.

Rejuvenation Strategies

To counteract these aging effects, several approaches can be considered:

1. Botulinum Toxin (Botox) for Brow Lift

Injecting botulinum toxin into specific muscles can provide a subtle lift to the eyebrows.

Procedure: Botox is injected into the muscles that pull the eyebrows downward, allowing the forehead muscles to lift the brows naturally.

Benefits: This non-invasive treatment can create a more open and refreshed eye area without surgery.

Considerations: Results are temporary, typically lasting 3 to 4 months, and maintenance treatments are necessary to sustain the effect.

2. Cosmetic Tattooing (Microblading)

For those with sparse or over-plucked eyebrows, cosmetic tattooing offers a semi-permanent solution.

Procedure: Microblading involves using fine needles to deposit pigment into the skin, creating the appearance of fuller, well-shaped eyebrows.

Benefits: This technique can restore the look of natural brows, enhancing facial symmetry and framing the eyes effectively.

Considerations: It's essential to choose a skilled and experienced technician to achieve natural-looking results. Regular touch-ups are required to maintain the desired appearance.

3. Eyebrow Growth Serums

Topical serums can promote eyebrow hair growth and improve density.

Application: Applied daily, these serums contain ingredients that stimulate hair follicles.

Benefits: Over time, users may notice thicker and fuller eyebrows.

Considerations: Results vary among individuals, and consistent use is necessary to see improvements.

4. Makeup Techniques

Utilizing makeup can provide an immediate enhancement to eyebrow appearance.

Application: Brow pencils, powders, and gels can fill in sparse areas, define shape, and add color to greying hairs.

Benefits: Makeup offers a non-permanent way to achieve the desired brow look, allowing for flexibility and daily adjustments.

Considerations: Proper application techniques are essential to achieve a natural appearance.

Maintaining well-groomed and appropriately shaped eyebrows is vital for facial balance and highlighting the eyes' beauty. Consulting with professionals in dermatology or cosmetic artistry can help determine the most suitable approach to rejuvenate and enhance the eyebrows, contributing to a more youthful and harmonious facial appearance..

Nita in 1970s over plucked eyebrows	2025 Eyebrows tattooed to restore more balanced shape for face
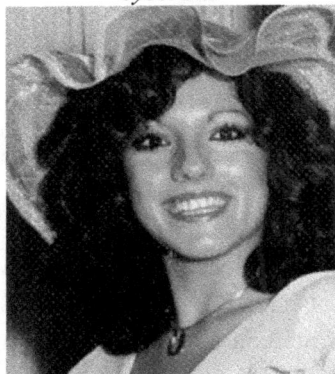	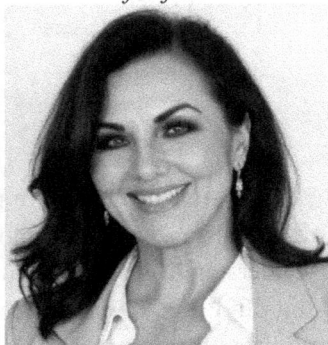

CHAPTER 26: AGING AND THINNING HAIR. UNDERSTANDING CAUSES AND EXPLORING TREATMENTS

Hair plays a significant role in personal identity and self-esteem. As individuals age, it is common to experience hair thinning and loss. Understanding the structure of hair, the reasons behind its thinning, and the available treatments can aid in managing and potentially mitigating these changes.

Structure of Hair

Each hair strand comprises two main parts:

1. Hair Shaft: The visible part above the skin's surface.

2. Hair Root: Located beneath the skin, housed within the hair follicle.

The hair shaft consists of three layers:

Cuticle: The outermost layer made of overlapping cells, protecting the inner layers.

Cortex: The middle layer containing keratin, providing strength, colour, and texture.

Medulla: The innermost layer, present in thicker hair strands, whose function is not fully understood.

Causes of Hair Thinning with Age

Several factors contribute to hair thinning as individuals age:

Hormonal Changes: Decreased estrogen levels in women during menopause and increased sensitivity to dihydrotestosterone (DHT) in both genders can lead to hair follicle miniaturization.

Genetics: A family history of hair loss increases the likelihood of experiencing similar patterns.

Thyroid Disorders: Both hyperthyroidism and hypothyroidism can disrupt the hair growth cycle, leading to thinning.

Reduced Blood Supply: Aging can lead to decreased circulation to hair follicles, impairing nutrient delivery and hair growth.

Nutritional Deficiencies: Lack of essential nutrients like iron, zinc, and vitamins can weaken hair structure.

Mechanical Stress: Hairstyles that pull hair tightly can cause traction alopecia, leading to receding hairlines.

Treatment Options

Various treatments are available to address hair thinning:

1. Platelet-Rich Plasma (PRP) Therapy

PRP involves injecting concentrated platelets from the patient's blood into the scalp to stimulate hair growth.

Procedure: Blood is drawn, processed to concentrate platelets, and injected into thinning areas.

Benefits: May promote hair growth and increase hair density.

Considerations: Multiple sessions are often required; results vary among individuals.

2. Mesotherapy

This technique involves injecting a mixture of vitamins, minerals, and medications into the scalp.

Procedure: Microinjections deliver nutrients directly to hair follicles.

Benefits: Aims to improve scalp health and stimulate hair growth.

Considerations: Effectiveness varies; multiple treatments may be necessary.

3. Exosome Therapy

A novel treatment using exosomes (small vesicles) to promote hair regeneration.

Procedure: Exosomes are injected into the scalp to encourage hair follicle activity.

Benefits: Potential to stimulate hair growth at the cellular level.

Considerations: Still under research; availability may be limited.

4. Low-Level Laser Therapy (LLLT) Caps

Devices that emit low-level lasers to stimulate hair follicles.

Procedure: Wearing a laser-emitting cap for a specified duration regularly.

Benefits: Non-invasive method to promote hair growth.

Considerations: Requires consistent use over time; results vary.

5. Scalp Micropigmentation (SMP)

A cosmetic tattooing technique to create the illusion of fuller hair.

Procedure: Pigment is applied to the scalp to mimic hair follicles.

Benefits: Provides the appearance of density in thinning areas.

Considerations: Does not promote hair growth; primarily aesthetic.

6. Topical Home Care

Incorporating specific products into daily routines can support hair health.

Options: Topical minoxidil, specialized shampoos, and conditioners.

Benefits: May slow hair loss and promote regrowth.

Considerations: Consistency is key; results may take months to appear.

Consulting with a dermatologist or hair specialist is essential to determine the most appropriate treatment based on individual needs and the underlying causes of hair thinning.

CHAPTER 27: BODY SKIN "HOW IT DIFFERS FROM FACIAL SKIN & EFFECTIVE TREATMENTS FOR REJUVENATION AND TIGHTENING"

Understanding the Structural Differences Between Facial and Body Skin

While the skin functions as a protective barrier throughout the body, its structure varies depending on location. The body's skin differs significantly from facial skin, influencing how it ages, heals, and responds to treatments.

1. Thickness

Body skin is generally thicker than facial skin, except in delicate areas like the eyelids.

The dermis on the body is denser, containing thicker collagen fibers, making it more resistant to external factors but slower to regenerate.

2. Collagen and Elasticity

Body skin has a lower cell turnover rate, meaning it renews more slowly than facial skin.

It contains fewer sebaceous glands, making it more prone to dryness and laxity over time.

3. Fat Distribution and Cellulite Formation

Facial fat is evenly distributed, maintaining smooth contours.

Body fat is compartmentalized within fibrous septae (connective tissue bands), which contribute to cellulite formation.

4. Healing and Regeneration

Facial skin heals faster due to its higher vascularization.

Body skin, especially in areas like the thighs and abdomen, has poorer circulation, leading to slower healing and collagen remodeling.

Cellulite : What Causes It?

Cellulite affects up to 90% of women and is caused by a combination of:

Fibrous septae pulling the skin downward, creating dimples.

Fat pushing between these bands, leading to a lumpy appearance.

Weakening of skin structure due to collagen loss and poor circulation.

Hormonal factors, especially estrogen, which influences fat storage and skin integrity.

Genetics, which determine skin thickness, elasticity, and fat distribution.

Because cellulite is not just a fat issue but a structural problem, traditional weight loss methods do not always help. Effective treatments must target the connective tissue, skin quality, and circulation to achieve visible improvement.

Advanced Treatments for Body Skin Rejuvenation and Tightening

Improving skin laxity, volume loss, and cellulite requires injectables, energy-based devices, regenerative treatments, and mechanical techniques.

1. Subcision for Cellulite Releasing Fibrous Septae with a Cannula

How it Works: A blunt-tip cannula is used to manually break the fibrous septae responsible for cellulite dimpling.

Why it's Important: Once released, the skin can smooth out naturally, reducing visible dimples.

Best for:

Deep, tethered cellulite

Prepping the skin for biostimulatory fillers like Sculptra

Combining with PRP to speed healing and collagen stimulation

2. Sculptra® Hyperdiluted Collagen Biostimulation

How it Works: Sculptra (poly-L-lactic acid) is a collagen stimulator that, when hyperdiluted, spreads over a large area to enhance skin thickness, elasticity, and volume.

Best for:

Crepey skin on arms, abdomen, thighs, and buttocks

Skin laxity and cellulite improvement

Combining with subcision to fill areas of volume loss

3. Radiesse® Hyperdiluted Immediate & Long-Term Tightening

How it Works: Radiesse (calcium hydroxylapatite) stimulates collagen while providing an immediate lifting effect. When hyperdiluted, it improves skin texture, hydration, and firmness.

Best for:

Décolletage rejuvenation

Knees, arms, and abdominal skin tightening

Smoothing skin after cellulite treatments

4. PRP (Platelet-Rich Plasma) : Regenerative Therapy

How it Works: PRP contains growth factors that stimulate collagen and elastin, improving skin renewal and tissue repair.

Best for:

Stretch marks and scarring

Post-subcision healing and enhanced skin tightening

Combination with microneedling or radiofrequency for deeper skin remodelling

5. Radiofrequency (RF) Thermal Skin Tightening

How it Works: RF energy heats the dermis, stimulating collagen contraction and gradual remodelling over time.

Best for:

Post-pregnancy skin tightening

Moderate laxity on the abdomen, arms, and thighs

Cellulite reduction (when paired with lymphatic drainage)

Popular RF Devices: Thermage®, Exilis®, Venus Legacy®

6. Ultherapy® Ultrasound-Based Deep Lifting

How it Works: Ultherapy delivers micro-focused ultrasound energy to stimulate collagen production at the SMAS layer (deep connective tissue).

Best for:

Tightening loose skin on arms, stomach, knees, and buttocks

Patients wanting a non-invasive lifting effect

7. Morpheus®: RF Micro needling for Deep Tissue Remodelling

How it Works: A combination of micro needling and RF energy penetrates deep into the skin and tightens underlying tissue.

Best for:

Crepey skin and mild volume loss on arms, abdomen, and thighs

Cellulite dimpling improvement

Long-term skin firming and collagen regeneration

Other Skin Tightening & Cellulite Reduction Technologies

Emsculpt Neo® Uses RF heating and high-intensity focused electromagnetic (HIFEM) stimulation to tighten skin and tone muscles. Ideal for abdomen, buttocks, and arms.

Velashape® A combination of infrared light, RF, and vacuum suction to improve cellulite and skin tone.

Carboxytherapy: Injecting CO2 gas under the skin to increase circulation and collagen production, improving cellulite and elasticity.

Endermologie® A mechanical massage therapy that enhances lymphatic drainage and stimulates fibroblasts to reduce cellulite.

Combining Treatments for Optimal Results

The best outcomes for body skin rejuvenation and cellulite reduction come from combining multiple treatments:

Subcision + Sculptra/Radiesse Breaking down fibrous bands, then adding collagen stimulation and volume.

Morpheus8 + PRP Combining microneedling, RF, and regenerative therapy for long-term firming.

Ultherapy + RF treatments Deep collagen activation paired with surface tightening.

Muscle stimulation (Emsculpt Neo) + skin tightening Enhancing underlying structure for better skin support.

Conclusion

Body skin differs from facial skin in its thickness, collagen structure, fat distribution, and ability to heal. These differences require specialized treatments to improve laxity, volume loss, and cellulite.

By incorporating a combination of injectables, regenerative therapies, and energy-based treatments, practitioners can offer their patients highly effective, long-lasting solutions for firmer, smoother, and more youthful-looking skin.

With the right approach, non-surgical skin tightening and cellulite reduction can deliver remarkable, natural-looking result helping patients achieve renewed confidence in their bodies.

3 Sessions of PRP with cannula

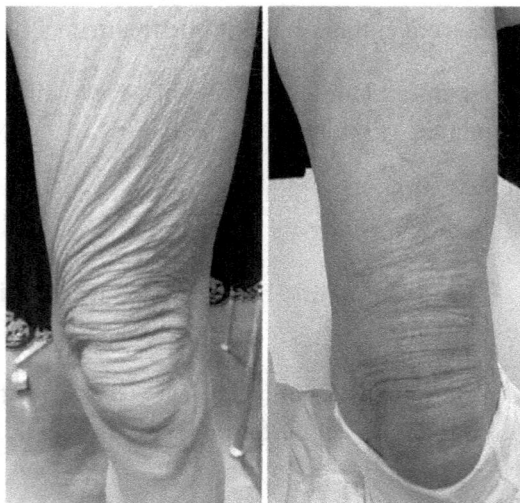

Chapter 28: Botulinum Toxin Type A What It Is, Manufacturing, Safety, and Variants

What Is Botulinum Toxin Type A?

Botulinum toxin type A is a purified neurotoxin derived from the Clostridium botulinum bacterium. It is important to note that Botox is NOT the bacterium itself rather, it is a highly refined neurotoxin that is carefully extracted, purified, and diluted to ensure safe medical and cosmetic use.

Botulinum Toxin vs. Clostridium Botulinum Bacteria

Clostridium botulinum is a naturally occurring bacterium found in soil, lakes, and forests.

This bacterium can produce botulinum toxin under certain conditions, such as low-oxygen environments.

The toxin is one of the most potent biological substances, capable of blocking nerve signals and causing paralysis in high doses.

In medicine, only a purified and controlled amount of botulinum toxin type A is used making it safe when administered correctly.

How Was Botulinum Toxin Discovered?

The first therapeutic use of botulinum toxin was pioneered in the 1970s by ophthalmologists Dr. Jean and Dr. Alastair Carruthers while treating eye muscle disorders (e.g., strabismus, blepharospasm). They observed that patients developed smoother skin in treated areas, leading to the cosmetic use of botulinum toxin. In 1991, the first botulinum toxin treatment for wrinkles was documented, and Botox® was officially approved for cosmetic use.

How Is Botox Manufactured?

The production of Botox (OnabotulinumtoxinA) involves a highly controlled, multi-step purification and testing process to ensure its safety and efficacy. The manufacturing process includes:

1. Culturing the Bacteria

The process begins with the controlled growth of Clostridium botulinum in a secure laboratory environment.

The bacterium is grown under strict conditions to allow it to naturally produce botulinum toxin type A.

2. Harvesting the Toxin

Once enough toxin is produced, the bacteria are removed, leaving only the botulinum toxin.

The toxin is carefully extracted and separated from other bacterial components.

3. Purification Process

The extracted botulinum toxin undergoes multiple purification steps to remove any unwanted proteins or contaminants.

This process ensures that only the pure, active botulinum toxin type A remains.

The purified toxin is then stabilized using human albumin, a protein that helps maintain its structure and effectiveness.

4. Dilution & Standardization

The purified botulinum toxin is diluted to an exact concentration to create the final medical-grade Botox product.

Each batch is rigorously tested to ensure potency, consistency, and safety.

The product is then packaged into vials and stored under strict temperature-controlled conditions to preserve its activity.

Why Is Botox Safe for Medical Use?

Although botulinum toxin in its natural form is highly toxic, the controlled doses used in Botox treatments are small, purified, and carefully measured for safety.

Extremely Low Doses: The amount of botulinum toxin used in medical treatments is millions of times lower than what would cause toxicity.

Purified & Stabilized: The purification process removes unnecessary bacterial components, ensuring only the active neurotoxin is present.

FDA & TGA Approved: Botox has been extensively studied and approved by regulatory agencies such as the U.S. FDA (Food and Drug Administration) and Australia's TGA

(Therapeutic Goods Administration) for both medical and cosmetic use.

Injected in Targeted Areas: Unlike botulism (which affects the whole body), Botox is administered in small, precise doses to specific muscles making it a safe and effective localized treatment.

Different Types of Botulinum Toxin Type A & Their Differences

There are now many different brands of botulinum toxin available worldwide, each with different formulations, carrier proteins, diffusion properties, and unit measurements.

Common FDA/TGA-Approved Brands and Their Differences

Brand	Protein Composition	Carrier/Base	Key Differences
Botox (Onabotulinum toxinA)	Has complexing proteins	Human albumin & saline	Most well-known, stable diffusion, predictable effects
Xeomin (Incobotulinum toxinA)	No accessory proteins (pure toxin)	Human albumin & saline	No complexing proteins = reduced risk of resistance
Dysport (Abobotulinum toxinA)	Has complexing proteins	Human albumin & lactose	Spreads more than Botox, good for larger areas
Jeuveau (Prabotulinumt oxinA)	Has complexing proteins	Human albumin & saline	Marketed as #Newtox in the U.S.
Revance Daxxify (Daxxibotulinu mtoxinA-lanm)	Peptide-stabilized (no human albumin)	Peptide-based carrier	Potentially longer-lasting results
Lytebo (Botulinum Toxin Type A, China-based)	Has complexing proteins	Glucose & gelatin	Newer product, limited international experience

Understanding units in Botulinum Toxin

A unit measures the toxin biological activity (its ability to block nerve signals).

However, units are NOT interchangeable between brands because each company uses a different potency assay.

Brand	Unit Conversion	Key Differences
Botox & Xeomin	1 Botox unit = 1 Xeomin unit	Direct unit-to-unit conversion
Dysport	2.5 Dysport units = 1 Botox unit	Dysport diffuses more, requiring more units for an equivalent effect
Jeuveau/Nuceiva	1:1 with Botox	Considered equivalent to Botox in dosing
Lytebo	Similar to Botox (research ongoing)	Limited data outside China
Daxxify	1:1 with Botox	Early studies suggest longer duration

WARNING: Counterfeit & Illegal Botulinum Toxin Products

Dangers of Fake or Unapproved Botulinum Toxin

Recent Incident in Sydney:

Three people were hospitalized with botulism poisoning after receiving botulinum toxin injections from an unlicensed backyard injector who bought fake products from the internet. Symptoms included severe muscle paralysis, difficulty breathing, and hospitalization.

How to Avoid Counterfeit Toxins

Only receive treatments from licensed medical professionals (doctors, registered nurses, trained aesthetic practitioners).

Ensure the clinic uses FDA- or TGA-approved brands. Avoid discount offers from non-reputable sources (e.g., home-based injectors, overseas imports). Check the packaging legitimate toxins come with lot numbers, expiration dates, and secure labeling. Do not buy toxins online,only licensed professionals can legally obtain these medications.

Conclusion

Botox is NOT the bacterium it is a purified, controlled form of botulinum toxin type A.

It is produced through a strict manufacturing process, ensuring safety, purity, and effectiveness. There are now many different brands on the market, each with unique properties, diffusion rates, and unit conversions.FDA/TGA-approved toxins include Botox, Xeomin, Dysport, Jeuveau, Lytebo, and Daxxify. Counterfeit and illegally imported toxins pose serious health risks, including botulism poisoning. Always seek treatment from a reputable clinic that uses licensed and approved botulinum toxin brands. Understanding the manufacturing, purification, and regulatory approval of Botox helps dispel myths and reinforces why choosing a qualified provider is essential for both safety and results.

Relfydess™: The New Tox on the Block

What is Relfydess™

Relfydess™ (RelabotulinumtoxinA) is a new botulinum toxin introduced by Galderma as an alternative to established brands like Botox®, Dysport®, Xeomin®, and Jeuveau®. It stands out due to its ready-to-use liquid formulation, a different botulinum strain, and potentially longer-lasting effects. Designed for facial wrinkle treatment, it offers fast-acting, consistent results while simplifying the preparation process for practitioners.

Key Differences of Relfydess™

1. Different Botulinum Strain

• Most neuromodulators (Botox, Dysport, Xeomin, Jeuveau) are derived from the Hall strain of Clostridium botulinum.

• Relfydess™ comes from a different botulinum strain, which may contribute to variations in diffusion, longevity, and resistance development.

2. Unit Measurement and Volume

• Relfydess™ uses the same unit measurement as Dysport®, meaning that the dose conversion will align with Dysport protocols.

• However, its injection volume matches Botox®, making it easier to transition for practitioners familiar with Botox's dilution and handling.

3. Ready-to-Use Liquid Formula

• Unlike Botox, Dysport, and Jeuveau, which come as a powder that requires reconstitution, Relfydess™ is pre-mixed in liquid form.

• This eliminates potential dilution errors, ensures consistent dosing, and streamlines the preparation process.

4. Potential for Faster Onset

• Botox and Xeomin typically take 3–5 days for visible results.

• Dysport has a faster onset (2–3 days) but diffuses more widely.

• Clinical studies suggest Relfydess™ may start working as early as Day 1 for some patients, making it one of the quickest-acting options available.

5. Duration of Effects

• Botox, Dysport, Xeomin, and Jeuveau generally last 3–4 months before retreatment is needed.

• Early data indicates Relfydess™ may last up to 6 months in some patients, potentially offering extended effectiveness.

Considerations for Practitioners and Patients
• For injectors, the pre-mixed formulation can reduce preparation time and improve consistency. However, those accustomed to Botox or Dysport may need to adjust unit conversions.

• For patients, Relfydess™ may offer a faster onset and longer duration, but individual results can vary.

• Since Relfydess™ uses a different botulinum strain, it may be an option for those who have developed resistance to other toxins.

How Relfydess™ Compares to Other Toxins.

Feature	Relfydess™	Botox® (Onabotulinumtoxina)	Dysport® (Abobotulinumtoxina)	Xeomin® (Incobotulinumtoxina)	Jeuveau® (Prabotulinumtoxina)
Botulinum Strain	Unique strain	*Hall strain	Hall strain	Hall strain (purified)	Hall strain
Formulation	Pre-mixed liquid	Powder (requires mixing)	Powder (requires mixing)	Powder (no complexing proteins)	Powder (requires mixing)
Onset of Action	As early as 1 day	3–5 days	2–3 days (faster spread)	3–4 days	3–4 days
Longevity	Up to 6 months	3–4 months	3–4 months	3–4 months	3–4 months
Spread/Diffusion	Balanced	Precise	More diffusion	Precise	Similar to Botox
Resistance Risk	Lower (unique strain)	Can develop resistance	Can develop resistance	Lower (no complexing proteins)	Can develop resistance
Unit Measurement	Same as Dysport	Botox units	Dysport units	Botox units	Botox units

* OnabotulinumtoxinA • The "Hall strain" is the original strain used by Dr. Edward J. Schantz in the 1940s for medical research and is still used in the production of Botox today.

Aesthetic Areas Treated and Injection Considerations with Botulinum Toxin A:

1. Forehead (Frontalis)

Goal: Smooth horizontal lines while maintaining brow position.

Care: Avoid injecting too low or too deep laterally — may drop brows or cause heavy eyelids.

Use light dosing across upper frontalis to preserve natural movement and lift.

2. Frown Lines (Glabellar Complex – Procerus & Corrugators)

Goal: Soften vertical "11" lines.

Care: Avoid injecting too deep into the central glabella near the supraorbital foramen — can affect levator palpebrae superioris, causing ptosis.

3. Crow's Feet (Orbicularis Oculi)

Goal: Soften lateral eye wrinkles.

Care: Avoid deep or low injection near zygomatic arch — may cause cheek shelving or heavy nasolabial folds.

4. Bunny Lines (Nasalis)

Goal: Reduce nasal scrunch lines.

Care: Avoid diffusion toward the levator labii superioris alaeque nasi — may drop the upper lip.

5. Lip Lines (Perioral)

Goal: Soften vertical lip lines.

Care: Over-treatment may elongate the top lip, distort smile or affect lip competence. Use microdoses.

6. DAO (Depressor Anguli Oris)

Goal: Upturn marionette area/downturned mouth corners.

Care: Avoid diffusion to depressor labii inferioris (DLI) — may cause crooked smile or lip drop.

7. Masseter Muscle

Goal: Facial slimming, treat bruxism or clenching.

Care: Avoid superior and anterior spread to risorius muscle — may impair smiling or cause flat expression.

8. Nose

Tip Lift: Microdose into depressor septi nasi to lift tip.

Narrowing: Target nasalis for gentle narrowing.

Hay Fever Relief: Intranasal injection may reduce symptoms (off-label).

9. Nefertiti Lift

Target: Lower face/jawline — platysma.

Goal: Sharpen jawline, reduce jowls.

Care: Correct dosing avoids weakening neck support.

10. Platysma Bands

Goal: Soften neck bands, improve neck profile.

Care: Over-treatment may affect swallowing or lifting the head.

11. Eyebrow Lifts

Medial Lift: Relax depressor supercilii (DSS).

Lateral Lift: Inject into lateral orbicularis or temporalis to elevate tail of brow.

Therapeutic & Advanced Uses:

12. Hyperhidrosis

Areas: Axillae, palms, soles, scalp.

Care: Treat one hand at a time to avoid bilateral weakness.

13. Trapezius Muscles

Goal: Slim upper shoulders for a more elegant neck profile.

14. Calf Slimming (Popular in Asia)

Target: Gastrocnemius.

Care: High doses required; avoid weakness in gait.

15. Mesotherapy (Micro-Botox)

Use: Superficial injections to reduce pore size, oil, and acne activity.

16. Bell's Palsy

Goal: Relax unaffected side to create facial symmetry.

Care: Requires expert anatomical precision and custom dosing.

Expected Results of Botulinum Toxin A Injection:

Onset: 3–5 days

Peak Effect: 10–14 days

Duration: 3–4 months on average (masseters and hyperhydrosis 7-9 months.)

CHAPTER 29: UNDERSTANDING DERMAL FILLERS: COMPOSITION, MANUFACTURING, AND RHEOLOGY

What Are Dermal Fillers?

Dermal fillers are gel-like substances injected beneath the skin to restore volume, smooth wrinkles, enhance facial contours, and hydrate the skin. Most modern dermal fillers are composed of hyaluronic acid (HA), a naturally occurring substance in the human body that retains moisture and adds plumpness to the skin. Unlike botulinum toxin (which relaxes muscles), fillers work by physically adding volume to areas that have lost structure due to aging or other factors.

Where Do Fillers Come From?

Modern HA fillers are made in laboratories through a process called bacterial fermentation. Special strains of Streptococcus bacteria are used to produce hyaluronic acid, which is then purified, cross-linked (to make it last longer in the skin), and turned into a smooth injectable gel.

Discovery of Dermal Fillers: Early fillers included collagen-based products derived from bovine (cow) sources, requiring allergy testing. In the late 1990s, scientists developed hyaluronic acid (HA) fillers, which were safer, more biocompatible, and longer-lasting.

Today, HA fillers are the most commonly used fillers worldwide due to their natural integration with human tissue and reversibility using the enzyme hyaluronidase.

Hyaluronic Acid in the Body

HA is a sugar molecule (glycosaminoglycan) found naturally in skin, joints, and connective tissues. It can hold up to 1,000 times its weight in water, making it a key molecule for skin hydration and volume retention. Our body naturally produces and degrades HA daily, with enzymes like hyaluronidase breaking it down within hours to days.

Why Do HA Fillers Last Longer?

Since natural HA degrades quickly, scientists developed synthetic modifications to make HA fillers last longer in the skin.

How Are HA Fillers Made?

The Manufacturing Process of HA Fillers

1. **Fermentation**: HA is synthesized through bacterial fermentation (typically using Streptococcus bacteria).

The HA is then purified and processed into a gel-like form.

2. **Crosslinking with BDDE**: To increase longevity, HA molecules are chemically crosslinked using 1,4-butanediol diglycidyl ether (BDDE).

BDDE acts as a binding agent, linking HA molecules together, preventing rapid degradation, and extending the fillers durability.

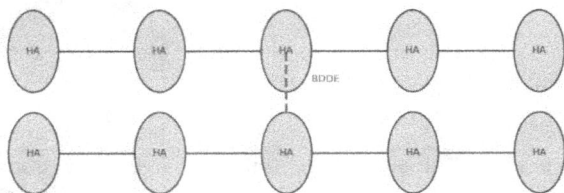

Chains of HA crosslinked with BDDE to increase longevity

3. **Customization of HA Fillers**: Different fillers are created by modifying the level of crosslinking, particle size, and gel consistency, producing different types suited for various treatments.

What Is BDDE?

BDDE (1,4-Butanediol Diglycidyl Ether) is a crosslinking agent used to stabilize HA in dermal fillers. Without BDDE, HA fillers would break down within days. The amount of BDDE and the crosslinking method determine how firm, elastic, and long-lasting the filler will be.

How Does Crosslinking Affect Longevity & Thickness?

The more crosslinking, the longer-lasting and firmer the filler:

Crosslinking Level	Filler Properties	Best Use Cases
Low Crosslinking	More fluid, hydrating, integrates easily	Skin boosters, superficial fine lines
Moderate Crosslinking	Balance of flexibility and structure	Lips, tear troughs, mid-face volume
High Crosslinking	Thick, firm, long-lasting	Cheeks, jawline, deep structural support

Different HA Filler Technologies & How They Work

PEG vs. BDDE Cross-Linking in Dermal Fillers: What's the Difference?

Most dermal fillers use hyaluronic acid (HA), but to make them last longer in the skin, the HA needs to be stabilized using a chemical cross-linking process. The traditional method uses BDDE (1,4-Butanediol Diglycidyl Ether), while a newer alternative is PEG (Polyethylene Glycol) cross-linking.

BDDE has been the standard for years and is safe for most people, but tiny traces of the chemical may remain in the filler after manufacturing. In rare cases, BDDE-based fillers can trigger inflammatory reactions or delayed nodules, especially in sensitive individuals.

PEG, on the other hand, is a medical-grade polymer known for its biocompatibility and low immune response. PEG-crosslinked fillers, such as Neauvia's range, have been designed to be BDDE-free, meaning they contain no epoxy-based crosslinkers. PEG-based fillers are reported to cause less swelling, lower risk of immune reactions, and smoother integration into the skin.

They also have a more elastic and flexible texture, making them ideal for natural-looking volume and movement.

Both BDDE and PEG fillers are safe and effective, but PEG cross-linking offers a purer, more advanced alternative with a lower risk of long-term complications.

Various filler brands have proprietary crosslinking technologies that influence their consistency, longevity, and integration.

PEG Cross-Linking in Dermal Fillers: Another HA Linking technology

Polyethylene Glycol (PEG) cross-linking is a modern advancement in dermal fillers, offering longer-lasting, more hydrating, and biocompatible results compared to traditional BDDE (1,4-butanediol diglycidyl ether) cross-linking. This technology creates a smooth, natural look with reduced risk of swelling or inflammation, making it ideal for delicate areas like under-eyes, lips, and hands.

Why Choose PEG Fillers?

Longer-Lasting – PEG stabilizes hyaluronic acid (HA) more effectively, slowing breakdown.

Superior Hydration – PEG fillers retain more water, improving skin plumpness.

Low Inflammation Risk – PEG is highly biocompatible, reducing sensitivity or swelling.

Soft, Natural Integration – Especially useful for areas requiring smooth transitions.

Fillers That Use PEG Technology

• **Neauvia Intense & Neauvia Stimulate** – Provides volume and stimulates collagen production.

• **Matex Lab HA Hydrogels** – A range of hydration-focused fillers for different facial areas.

• **Novel PEGDE-HA 24** – Specifically designed for natural lip enhancement with minimal swelling.

Filler Technologies Explained

When it comes to dermal fillers, not all hyaluronic acid (HA) gels are created equal. The way the HA is crosslinked and structured affects how the filler behaves — its softness, longevity, lift capacity, and integration into tissue. Here's a breakdown of some of the most widely used proprietary technologies in today's top fillers:

1. Vycross Technology (Allergan – Juvederm Voluma, Volbella, Volift, etc.)

• What it is: A blend of low and high molecular weight HA, crosslinked together using BDDE.

• Why it matters: The low-weight HA allows for tighter crosslinking, making the gel smoother and longer-lasting.

• Designed to integrate well with tissue and give natural volume with minimal swelling.

• Voluma is firmer for cheeks and structure, while Volbella is softer for lips and fine lines.

• Bonus: High moldability and durability with fewer lumps.

2. Hyalocross Technology (Allergan – Juvederm Ultra and Ultra Plus)

• What it is: An earlier generation technology that uses only high molecular weight HA, crosslinked with BDDE.

• Why it matters: Gives a more gel-like consistency, slightly more water-attracting (hydrophilic), so more swelling than Vycross.

- Good for volumizing lips or nasolabial folds, but doesn't last as long as Vycross fillers.

- Still widely used due to its proven performance and affordability.

3. RHA (Resilient Hyaluronic Acid – Teoxane RHA 1–4)

- What it is: HA that is minimally crosslinked and processed gently to preserve its natural long-chain structure.

- Why it matters: Moves dynamically with facial expressions, making it ideal for lips, perioral lines, and dynamic areas.

- Designed to mimic natural HA more closely, offering a soft, elastic feel.

- RHA 4 is great for structure, while RHA 1 and 2 are better for fine lines and lips.

4. CPM (Cohesive Polydensified Matrix – Belotero by Merz)

- What it is: A unique crosslinking process that creates zones of varying density within the filler gel.

- Why it matters: Allows the filler to integrate seamlessly into tissue, minimizing the risk of lumps or Tyndall effect.

- Belotero Balance is so fine it can be used in the superficial dermis.

- Excellent for tear troughs, fine lines, and blending into delicate areas.

5. OBT (Optimal Balance Technology – Restylane Refyne, Defyne, etc. by Galderma)

- What it is: A crosslinking technique balancing HA size, flexibility, and support for natural facial movement.

- Why it matters: Designed to offer flexibility in motion while still lifting and contouring.

- Refyne is softer and better for moderate lines, while Defyne gives more structure for deeper folds.

- The structure allows strong support with stretch, making it ideal for smile lines and mobile areas.

6. NASHA® (Non-Animal Stabilized Hyaluronic Acid) was the first hyaluronic acid (HA) filler technology used in aesthetics. Developed for the Restylane® range, it uses a unique sieving process that filters the gel into uniform particle sizes, creating a structured, cohesive gel.

This makes it ideal for precise placement, contouring, and lifting—perfect for areas like the nasolabial folds, cheeks, and lips. Fillers made with NASHA® include Restylane® Classic, Restylane® Lyft, and Restylane® Vital.

Unlike other technologies that offer soft, flexible gels for dynamic movement (like OBT/XpresHAn or RHA®), NASHA® fillers are firmer and hold their shape.

This structure gives greater control for sculpting and definition, making them a go-to for injectors seeking predictable, long-lasting results with minimal migration.

Common HA Filler Technologies

Technology	Manufacturer	Properties	Best Used For
Vycross®	Juvederm (Allergan)	Small and large HA molecules mixed for smooth integration	Lips, under-eye, cheeks
Hylacross®	Juvederm (Allergan)	Larger, more structured HA chains	Nasolabial folds, volumization
Resilient Hyaluronic Acid (RHA®)	Teoxane	More elastic, moves with facial expressions	Dynamic areas (lips, nasolabial folds)
Cohesive Polydensified Matrix	Belotero (Merz)	Highly adaptable, integrates well	Fine lines, tear troughs
OBT (Optimal Balance Technology)	Restylane (Galderma)	Balanced crosslinking, adaptable texture	Mid-face, lips, contouring
Nasha	Restylane (Galderma)	Structured, firm, mouldable precise	Chin, jaw, cheeks, lips
Cold X (Cold cross linking)	Hugal	Low temp cross linking for purity and homogeneity	Cheeks, lips, perioral area
Ultra High Flexibility	QT Fillers/ BioPlus	Very elastic HA gel for high mobility areas	Perioral area, lips, tear troughs
Ariessence (Advanced HA technology)	Koru Pharmaceuticals	Lightweight gel with high moldability, balanced elasticity and cohesiveness	Lips, tear troughs,

Each brand modifies its crosslinking and particle size to create fillers tailored to different facial areas.

Rheology: Understanding the Properties of Fillers

Why Rheology Matters in Filler Selection

Rheology is the study of how a filler behaves under pressure and movement. It helps clinicians choose the right filler for the right area.

Key Rheological Properties of Fillers

Property	Meaning	Importance in Treatment
(Gel Elasticity or Stiffness)	Higher G= firmer filler, lower G = softer filler	High G cheeks, jawline; Low G = lips, under-eye
Viscosity	How thick or fluid the filler is	Higher viscosity = better volume support
Cohesivity	How well the filler holds together	High cohesivity = better lift, low cohesivity = smooth integration
Elasticity (Stretchability)	Ability to move with facial expressions	High elasticity = ideal for dynamic areas like lips

Example:

Cheekbone augmentation needs a filler with high G prime (firm structure) like Restylane Lyft or Juvederm Voluma

Lips require a softer, more flexible filler with moderate elasticity, like RHA 2 or Juvederm Volbella.

Skin Boosters: Hydration Without Structure

Unlike dermal fillers used for volume, skin boosters have minimal crosslinking, allowing them to spread easily and deeply hydrate the skin.

What Makes Skin Boosters Different?

Instead of lifting or contouring, skin boosters improve hydration, elasticity, and skin texture.

They are microinjected into the dermis, not deep like traditional fillers.

Skin boosters stimulate collagen production and moisture retention, creating glowing, plump skin.

Popular Skin Boosters:

Profhilo® (NAHYCO® technology hybrid HA molecules)

Juvederm Volite, Restylane Skinboosters, Teosyal Redensity

Choosing the Right Filler for Each Area

A skilled injector must select the correct filler based on:

The treatment area (e.g., deep structure vs. superficial hydration)

The patient's skin type and movement dynamics

The desired longevity and integration

Area	Recommended Filler Type
Cheeks & Jawline	High G prime (firm, lifting) Allergan Voluma, Volux Restylane Lyft Teoxane Ultra Deep
Tear Troughs (Under Eyes)	Low G prime™ (soft, hydrating) Belotero Balance, Teoxane Redensity 2
Lips	Moderate elasticity Teoxane RHA 2, Allergan Juvederm Volbella are for a natural look. Higher G prime is chosen for more defined fuller lips.
Nasolabial Folds	Medium viscosity Restylane Defyne, or Volyme. Juvederm Ultra
Skin Hydration (No Volume)	Skin boosters Profhilo, Volite

Conclusion

Dermal fillers are primarily made of hyaluronic acid (HA), a natural substance in the body. HA is broken down quickly, so crosslinking with BDDE is used to extend its longevity.

The more crosslinking, the thicker and longer-lasting the filler. Different brands use proprietary crosslinking technologies to modify filler behavior.

Rheology determines which filler is best suited for specific facial areas. Skin boosters, with minimal crosslinking, are designed for hydration rather than volume.

By understanding filler properties, technology, and rheology, clinicians can achieve safe, natural-looking, and long-lasting results tailored to each patient's needs.

Nita's filler preference guide for specific areas.

Area	Method	Juvederm	Restylane	Teoxane	Beletoro	Stylage	Artefiller
Forehead	Deep inj or canula	Volift	Refyne	RHA 3	Balance	S,M	Finelines
Temple	Deep inj or canula	Voluma	Volyme	Ultra deep	Volume	M, L,XL	Volume
Zygoma	Deep inj	Volux or voluma	Defyne, volyme	Ultra deep	Intense	L, XL, XXL	Volume
Pre Auricular	canula	Voluma or volift	Volyme	RHA 4	Volume	M, L	Volume
Malar	Deep inj	Volift or voluma	Volyme	RHA 4	Volume	L, XL	Volume
Naso Labial Folds	canula	Voluma or juvederm plus	Volyme	RHA 4 or ultra deep	Volume	L, XL	Universal
Pyriform fossa	Deep inj	Voluma or volux	Defyne	Ultra deep	Intense	XL, XXL	Volume
Nose	Deep inj bridge or canula	Juvederm ultra plus	Lyft	Ultra deep	Intense	XL	Volume
Lips	Canula or injection above muscle	Juvederm ultraplus, ultra, volift, vobella	Refine, restylane, volyme	RHA 3, KISS	Shape, contour, balance	S, M, L	Soft, lips
Marionette	Canula or needle	Voluma, juv plus, volift	Volyme	RHA 4	Volume	L, XL	Universal
Top lip lines	Canula or needle	Volift, vobella	Refyne	Rha 3 , Redensity 2	Balance	S	Soft
chin	Canula or deep inj	Voluma, volux	Defyne, lyft	Ultra deep	Intense	XL, XXL	Volume
Jaw	canula	Volux	Defyne, lyft	Ultra deep	Intense	XXL	Volume
Pre Jowl sulcus	Deep inj	Voluma, volux, ultra plus,	Volyme, defyne , lyft	Ultra deep	Volume	XL, XXL	Volume
Tear Troughs	canula	Vobella	Refyne, lyft (deep)	Redensity 2	Balance or soft	S, M	
Lines wrinkles	Superficial inj	Vobella	Refyne	Redensity 2	Balance or soft	S	Fine lines
Hands	Canula or needle inj	Juvederm ultra, volite	Skin booster	Redensity 1	Balance	L	

CHAPTER 30: FILLER BRANDS AND THERE RANGES

Restylane® (Galderma)

Restylane® is one of the world's most established and extensively researched dermal filler brands, manufactured by Galderma. It was the first hyaluronic acid (HA) filler to receive FDA approval and has been used globally for over two decades.

What sets Restylane apart is its diverse product portfolio, designed to treat different facial layers, movement patterns, and aesthetic concerns — from deep structural support to delicate skin quality improvement.

Restylane® Technologies Explained

Understanding the technology behind the gel is essential, as it determines how the filler behaves once injected.

1. NASHA™ Technology

(Non-Animal Stabilized Hyaluronic Acid)

- Produces firmer, more particulate gels

- Minimal swelling

- Excellent lifting capacity and projection

- Best suited to structural support and deep injections

Key Characteristics

- High G' (firmness)

- Sharp definition

- Stable shape over time

- Lower water attraction → less post-treatment swelling

2. OBT™ / XpresHAn™ Technology

(Optimal Balance Technology)

- Designed to move naturally with facial expressions
- Softer, more elastic gels
- Ideal for dynamic areas of the face

Key Characteristics

- Balanced firmness and flexibility
- Adapts to facial movement
- Smooth integration into tissue
- Natural-looking results at rest and in motion

The Complete Restylane® Range

Products, Technology & Indications

Restylane Lyft®

Technology: NASHA™

Indications

- Cheek augmentation
- Midface volume restoration
- Jawline contouring
- Structural support
- Age-related volume loss

Key Features

- Firm, lifting gel

- Excellent for deep supraperiosteal placement

- Provides strong projection and contour

Best for: Patients with significant volume loss or needing strong foundational support.

Restylane Defyne®

Technology: XpresHAn™

Indications

- Nasolabial folds

- Marionette lines

- Chin shaping

- Lower face support with movement

Key Features

- Supports facial expressions without stiffness

- Excellent balance of strength and flexibility

Best for: Patients with expressive faces who need structure without rigidity.

Restylane Refyne®

Technology: XpresHAn™

Indications

- Mild to moderate nasolabial folds

- Perioral lines

- Smile lines

Key Features

- Softer than Defyne
- Allows subtle correction
- Maintains natural animation

Best for: Early ageing or patients seeking subtle refinement.

Restylane Volyme®

Technology: NASHA™

Indications

- Cheek volumisation
- Facial contouring
- Structural midface support

Key Features

- High lifting power
- Long-lasting volume
- Excellent cheek projection

Best for: Midface rejuvenation and contour enhancement.

Restylane Kysse®

Technology: XpresHAn™

Indications

- Lip augmentation
- Lip definition
- Lip hydration

- Perioral lines

Key Features

- Designed specifically for lips

- Soft, flexible, kissable texture

- Maintains natural lip movement

Best for: Patients wanting natural, expressive lips without stiffness.

Restylane Silk®

Technology: NASHA™

Indications

- Fine perioral lines

- Smoker's lines

- Subtle lip enhancement

- Tear troughs (experienced injectors only)

Key Features

- Very fine particle size

- Smooth integration in delicate areas

Best for: Fine line correction and precision work.

Restylane Eyelight®

Technology: NASHA™

Indications

- Tear trough correction

- Under-eye hollows

Key Features

- Specifically designed for the infraorbital region
- Low swelling profile
- High safety margin when used correctly

Best for: Patients with under-eye volume loss and hollowing.

Restylane Skinboosters™

(Vital & Vital Light)

Technology: NASHA™

Indications

- Skin hydration
- Texture improvement
- Fine lines
- Crepey skin

Key Features

- Micro-droplet placement
- Improves skin quality rather than volume
- Enhances glow and elasticity

Best for: Patients seeking skin rejuvenation without altering facial shape.

Restylane Volyme + Lidocaine

Same indications as Volyme with enhanced comfort.

Clinical Considerations

- All Restylane products use non-animal HA

- HA is fully reversible with hyaluronidase

- Products vary in G', elasticity, and particle size

- Correct product selection + anatomical knowledge is critical to safety and results

Summary Table

Product	Technology	Primary Use
Lyft	NASHA	Structural lift, cheeks, jawline
Volyme	NASHA	Midface volume
Defyne	XpresHAn	Deep folds with movement
Refyne	XpresHAn	Moderate folds
Kysse	XpresHAn	Lips
Silk	NASHA	Fine lines
Eyelight	NASHA	Tear trough
Skinboosters	NASHA	Skin quality

Allergan Aesthetics – JUVÉDERM® Collection

Allergan Aesthetics, an AbbVie company, is one of the most recognised global leaders in medical aesthetics. The JUVÉDERM® range is among the most widely used hyaluronic acid (HA) fillers worldwide and is known for its smooth gel consistency, longevity, and predictable outcomes.

Juvederm fillers are designed to address volume loss, contouring, facial shaping, and skin quality, with different products tailored to specific facial depths and aesthetic goals.

Juvederm® Technologies Explained

All Juvederm fillers are based on proprietary cross-linking technologies that determine how the gel behaves in tissue.

1. Hylacross™ Technology

- Earlier Juvederm technology
- Uses highly cross-linked HA chains of uniform molecular weight
- Produces a smooth, cohesive gel
- High water affinity → more hydration and volume

Key Characteristics

- Smooth consistency
- Strong volumising effect
- Softer lift compared to Vycross
- Slightly higher swelling potential

Best suited for: Lips, superficial to mid-dermal volume correction, soft contouring.

2. Vycross™ Technology

- Advanced Allergan technology
- Combines low- and high-molecular-weight HA
- Requires less HA to achieve structure
- Results in longer-lasting, more efficient gels

Key Characteristics

- Greater longevity
- Less post-treatment swelling

- Smooth tissue integration

- Strong lift with natural contours

Best suited for: Structural support, contouring, deep and mid-face volumisation, jawline and chin.

The Juvederm® Range

Products, Technology & Indications

Juvederm Voluma® XC

Technology: Vycross™

Indications

- Cheek augmentation

- Midface volume loss

- Chin projection

- Structural facial contouring

Key Features

- High lifting capacity

- Excellent projection

- Long duration (up to 18–24 months in some patients)

Best for: Foundational support and facial reshaping.

Juvederm Volift® XC

(Also known as Juvederm Vollure® in some markets)

Technology: Vycross™

Indications

- Nasolabial folds

- Marionette lines

- Cheeks

- Jawline refinement

Key Features

- Balance of lift and flexibility

- Softer than Voluma

- Integrates well in dynamic areas

Best for: Moderate volume loss where movement matters.

Juvederm Volbella® XC

Technology: Vycross™

Indications

- Lips (subtle enhancement)

- Perioral lines

- Tear troughs (experienced injectors only)

Key Features

- Low G'

- Soft, spreadable gel

- Minimal swelling

- Excellent for delicate areas

Best for: Refinement rather than volume.

Juvederm Ultra® Range

(Ultra 2, 3, 4)

Technology: Hylacross™

Indications

- Lips

- Nasolabial folds

- Marionette lines

- Moderate volume replacement

Key Features

- Smooth, hydrating gels

- Softer feel

- Shorter longevity than Vycross range

Best for: Patients wanting softness, hydration, and flexibility.

Juvederm Ultra Plus®

Technology: Hylacross™

Indications

- Deeper folds

- Volume replacement

- Facial contouring

Key Features

- More robust than Ultra

- Higher lifting capacity

- Noticeable volumising effect

Best for: Moderate to deeper wrinkles with volume loss.

Juvederm Volux®

Technology: Vycross™

Indications

- Jawline definition
- Chin enhancement
- Lower face contouring

Key Features

- Highest G' in the Juvederm range
- Strong structural support
- Excellent shape retention

Best for: Lower face sculpting and definition.

Juvederm Volite®

Technology: Vycross™

Indications

- Skin hydration
- Texture improvement
- Fine lines
- Crepey skin

Key Features

- Skin booster, not a volumiser
- Micro-droplet technique
- Improves elasticity, glow, and smoothness
- Long-lasting skin quality improvement (up to 9 months)

Best for: Patients seeking skin rejuvenation without changing facial shape.

Clinical Considerations

- Juvederm fillers have high HA concentration
- Strong water-binding capacity → excellent hydration
- All products are reversible with hyaluronidase
- Product choice must consider:
    - Facial movement
    - Tissue depth
    - Desired lift vs softness
    - Risk areas (especially tear troughs and lips)

Summary Table

Product	Technology	Primary Use
Voluma	Vycross	Cheeks, chin, structure
Volift / Vollure	Vycross	Folds, cheeks, jawline
Volbella	Vycross	Lips, tear trough, fine lines
Volux	Vycross	Jawline, chin
Ultra	Hylacross	Lips, folds
Ultra Plus	Hylacross	Deeper folds
Volite	Vycross	Skin quality.

TEOSYAL® (Teoxane Laboratories, Switzerland)

TEOSYAL® is a premium Swiss hyaluronic acid (HA) dermal filler range developed by Teoxane Laboratories, a company known for its strong focus on rheology, safety, and tissue integration.

Teosyal fillers are widely respected for their purity, predictability, and broad product selection, allowing injectors to tailor treatments precisely to facial anatomy, movement, and skin quality.

Teosyal® Technologies Explained

Teosyal fillers are produced using proprietary cross-linking technologies that influence firmness, elasticity, and integration into tissue.

1. RHA® Technology

(Resilient Hyaluronic Acid)

- Designed to adapt to facial movement
- Mimics the natural behaviour of HA in youthful skin
- Maintains softness while providing structure

Key Characteristics

- High stretch and resilience
- Natural expression at rest and in motion
- Excellent integration in dynamic areas
- Reduced stiffness during facial animation

Best suited for: Dynamic facial areas where movement and expression are critical.

2. Preserved Network Technology

- Maintains the long-chain HA structure

- Results in smooth, cohesive gels

- Minimal chemical modification of HA

Key Characteristics

- High purity

- Predictable behaviour

- Good longevity

- Excellent safety profile

Best suited for: Structural support, volume restoration, and contouring.

The TEOSYAL® Range

Products, Technology & Indications

Teosyal RHA® 1

Technology: RHA®

Indications

- Fine lines

- Perioral lines

- Superficial wrinkles

- Skin texture refinement

Key Features

- Very soft and flexible

- Maintains natural facial expressions

Best for: Early ageing and subtle corrections.

Teosyal RHA® 2

Technology: RHA®

Indications

- Moderate wrinkles
- Nasolabial folds
- Marionette lines

Key Features

- Balance of softness and support
- Adapts well to movement

Best for: Dynamic mid-face wrinkles.

Teosyal RHA® 3

Technology: RHA®

Indications

- Deeper wrinkles
- Nasolabial folds
- Facial contouring

Key Features

- Greater lifting capacity
- Still flexible during expression

Best for: Advanced folds in expressive faces.

Teosyal RHA® 4

Technology: RHA®

Indications

- Cheek volume restoration
- Jawline support
- Facial contouring

Key Features

- Highest firmness in RHA range
- Strong structural support with movement adaptability

Best for: Dynamic contouring and volumisation.

Teosyal Ultra Deep®

Technology: Preserved Network

Indications

- Cheeks
- Chin projection
- Jawline sculpting
- Deep volume restoration

Key Features

- Very high G'
- Strong lifting and projection
- Excellent shape retention

Best for: Structural foundation and facial framework.

Teosyal Global Action®

Technology: Preserved Network

Indications

- Moderate to deep wrinkles
- Nasolabial folds
- Marionette lines

Key Features

- Balanced firmness
- Good durability
- Smooth tissue integration

Best for: Classic wrinkle correction.

Teosyal Kiss®

Technology: Preserved Network

Indications

- Lip augmentation
- Lip definition
- Perioral lines

Key Features

- Soft yet structured
- Natural lip movement
- Smooth feel

Best for: Natural lip enhancement.

Teosyal Redensity I®

Technology: Preserved Network + Dermal Redensification Complex

Indications

- Skin hydration
- Texture improvement
- Fine lines
- Dull skin

Key Features

- HA combined with amino acids, antioxidants, minerals, and vitamins
- Improves skin quality without volume

Best for: Skin revitalisation and glow.

Teosyal Redensity II®

Technology: Preserved Network

Indications

- Tear trough correction
- Under-eye hollows

Key Features

- Low swelling formulation
- Designed specifically for the infraorbital area
- Excellent safety profile when used correctly

Best for: Delicate under-eye rejuvenation.

Clinical Considerations

- Teosyal fillers are high-purity, non-animal HA
- All products are reversible with hyaluronidase

- RHA range is ideal for highly expressive patients

Product choice should consider:

- o Facial movement

- o Tissue depth

- o Desired projection vs flexibility

- o Risk zones (tear trough, lips)

Summary Table

Product	Technology	Primary Use
RHA 1	RHA	Fine lines
RHA 2	RHA	Moderate wrinkles
RHA 3	RHA	Deep folds
RHA 4	RHA	Dynamic contouring
Ultra Deep	Preserved Network	Structural volume
Global Action	Preserved Network	Wrinkle correction
Kiss	Preserved Network	Lips
Redensity I	PN + Dermal Complex	Skin quality
Redensity II	PN	Tear trough

NEAUVIA® (Matex Lab, Switzerland / Italy

NEAUVIA® is a next-generation hyaluronic acid (HA) dermal filler range developed by Matex Lab, combining Swiss precision with Italian innovation. What distinguishes Neauvia from many traditional fillers is its PEG-crosslinking technology and the inclusion of amino acids in selected products, positioning it at the intersection of structural filler and biostimulation.

Neauvia fillers are designed to provide strong structural support, excellent tissue integration, reduced inflammatory response, and long-term skin quality improvement.

Neauvia® Technologies Explained

1. PEG Cross-Linking Technology

(Polyethylene Glycol)

Unlike traditional BDDE cross-linking, Neauvia uses PEG, a biocompatible polymer widely used in medical devices.

Key Advantages

- High biocompatibility
- Lower inflammatory response
- Increased gel stability
- Improved longevity
- Reduced risk of delayed hypersensitivity reactions

Clinical Benefit: PEG creates a strong yet flexible HA network that integrates smoothly into tissue while maintaining structural integrity.

2. Amino Acid Enrichment

(Specific products only)

Certain Neauvia fillers are enriched with glycine and L-proline, essential building blocks for collagen synthesis.

Key Advantages

- Supports fibroblast activity
- Encourages collagen production

- Provides a biostimulatory effect beyond volume

Clinical Benefit: Improves skin quality, elasticity, and firmness over time.

The NEAUVIA® Range

Products, Technology & Indications

Neauvia Intense®

Technology: PEG-crosslinked HA

Indications

- Cheek volumisation
- Jawline contouring
- Chin projection
- Deep structural support

Key Features

- Very high G'
- Strong lifting and projection
- Excellent shape retention

Best for: Foundational facial framework and contouring.

Neauvia Intense Lips®

Technology: PEG-crosslinked HA

Indications

- Lip augmentation
- Lip contouring

- Lip hydration

Key Features

- Soft yet supportive gel
- Natural lip movement
- Reduced swelling profile

Best for: Natural-looking lips with definition and softness.

Neauvia Intense Rheology®

Technology: PEG-crosslinked HA

Indications

- Midface volume restoration
- Nasolabial folds
- Facial contouring

Key Features

- Optimised balance of elasticity and firmness
- Adapts well to dynamic areas

Best for: Areas requiring both support and movement.

Neauvia Stimulate®

Technology: PEG-crosslinked HA + Amino Acids

Indications

- Facial volume loss
- Skin laxity
- Collagen depletion

Key Features

- Biostimulatory filler

- Supports collagen production

- Gradual skin quality improvement

Best for: Patients with ageing skin needing structure plus regeneration.

Neauvia Hydro Deluxe®

Technology: PEG-crosslinked HA + Amino Acids

Indications

- Skin hydration

- Texture improvement

- Fine lines

- Crepey skin

Key Features

- Skin booster, not a volumiser

- Improves elasticity and glow

- Long-lasting hydration

Best for: Skin rejuvenation without volume change.

Neauvia Flux®

Technology: PEG-crosslinked HA

Indications

- Superficial wrinkles

- Fine lines

- Tear troughs (experienced injectors only)

Key Features

- Low G'

- Smooth, spreadable gel

- Minimal swelling

Best for: Delicate areas and fine corrections.

Neauvia Organic Intense®

Technology: PEG-crosslinked HA (High purity, organic origin)

Indications

- Structural volumisation

- Facial contouring

Key Features

- Extremely high purity HA

- Strong lifting capacity

- Excellent tissue integration

Best for: Patients requiring robust support with excellent tolerability.

Clinical Considerations

- PEG technology offers enhanced biocompatibility

- Reduced inflammatory and oedema profile

- All Neauvia fillers are reversible with hyaluronidase

- Amino-acid enriched products provide added biostimulation

- Ideal for patients concerned about:
    - Longevity
    - Tissue tolerance
    - Skin quality improvement alongside volume

Summary Table

Product	Technology	Primary Use
Intense	PEG	Structural volume
Intense Lips	PEG	Lip enhancement
Intense Rheology	PEG	Dynamic contouring
Stimulate	PEG + Amino Acids	Biostimulation
Hydro Deluxe	PEG + Amino Acids	Skin quality
Flux	PEG	Fine lines
Organic Intense	PEG	High-strength

Merz Aesthetics – Belotero® & Radiesse®

Merz Aesthetics is a global medical aesthetics company headquartered in Germany, known for its science-driven, anatomy-respecting approach to facial rejuvenation. Unlike some companies that focus solely on hyaluronic acid (HA) fillers, Merz offers both HA fillers and biostimulatory fillers, allowing practitioners to address volume, contour, structure, and collagen stimulation.

Merz's injectable portfolio centres around two flagship ranges:

- Belotero® – Hyaluronic acid fillers

- Radiesse® – Calcium hydroxylapatite (CaHA) biostimulatory filler

Merz® Technologies Explained

CPM® Technology

(Cohesive Polydensified Matrix)

Used in the Belotero® HA range

CPM technology creates a homogeneous, cohesive HA gel with varying densities within the same syringe.

Key Characteristics

- Smooth, uniform integration

- Minimal palpability

- Reduced risk of Tyndall effect

- Excellent tissue spread

Clinical Benefit: Allows fillers to integrate seamlessly into superficial and mid-dermal layers, producing soft, natural results, especially in delicate areas.

CaHA Microsphere Technology

Used in Radiesse®

Radiesse is composed of calcium hydroxylapatite microspheres suspended in a gel carrier.

Key Characteristics

- Immediate structural support

- Long-term collagen stimulation

- Biostimulatory rather than hydrophilic

- Non-HA filler (not reversible with hyaluronidase)

Clinical Benefit: Improves skin firmness, thickness, and elasticity over time while providing immediate contouring.

The BELOTERO® Range

Hyaluronic Acid Fillers

Belotero Balance®

Technology: CPM®

Indications

- Fine to moderate lines

- Perioral lines

- Tear troughs (experienced injectors only)

- Superficial wrinkles

Key Features

- Soft, smooth gel

- Excellent superficial integration

- Minimal Tyndall risk

Best for: Delicate areas and fine line correction.

Belotero Intense®

Technology: CPM®

Indications

- Nasolabial folds
- Marionette lines
- Moderate to deep wrinkles

Key Features

- Greater lifting capacity than Balance
- Maintains smooth tissue integration

Best for: Wrinkle correction requiring more support without stiffness.

Belotero Volume®

Technology: CPM®

Indications

- Cheek volumisation
- Midface volume loss
- Facial contouring

Key Features

- Higher G'
- Strong yet smooth projection
- Natural contouring

Best for: Midface rejuvenation and volume restoration.

Belotero Lips®

Technology: CPM®

Indications

- Lip augmentation
- Lip definition
- Perioral lines

Key Features

- Designed specifically for lips
- Soft, flexible, natural feel
- Good hydration

Best for: Natural, soft lip enhancement.

Belotero Revive®

Technology: CPM® + Glycerol

Indications

- Skin hydration
- Texture improvement
- Fine lines

Key Features

- Skin booster rather than volumiser
- Improves elasticity and glow
- Enhances skin quality without altering facial shape

Best for: Patients seeking skin rejuvenation rather than volume.

The RADIESSE® Range

Biostimulatory Fillers

Radiesse®

Composition: Calcium Hydroxylapatite (CaHA)

Indications

- Jawline contouring
- Cheek support
- Chin projection
- Lower face lifting
- Hand rejuvenation

Key Features

- Immediate lift and contour
- Long-term collagen stimulation
- Improves skin thickness and firmness
- Results may last 12–18 months or longer

Best for: Structural support and collagen regeneration.

Radiesse® (+)

(With lidocaine)

Same indications as Radiesse®, with improved patient comfort.

Diluted / Hyperdiluted Radiesse®

(Advanced injector technique)

Indications

- Skin laxity
- Crepey skin
- Neck, décolletage
- Arms, abdomen, knees, buttocks

Key Features

- Acts as a pure biostimulator
- Improves skin quality and firmness
- No volumisation when diluted appropriately

Best for: Skin tightening and collagen stimulation.

Clinical Considerations

- Belotero products are HA and reversible
- Radiesse is non-HA and not reversible
- Radiesse should not be used in lips or tear troughs
- Product selection must consider:
    o Desired volume vs stimulation
    o Reversibility
    o Skin thickness and laxity
    o Anatomical risk zones

Summary Tables

Belotero®

Product	Technology	Primary Use
Balance	CPM	Fine lines
Intense	CPM	Moderate–deep wrinkles
Volume	CPM	Cheek volume
Lips	CPM	Lips
Revive	CPM + Glycerol	Skin quality

Radiesse®

Product	Composition	Primary Use
Radiesse	CaHA	Structure & collagen
Radiesse (+)	CaHA + Lidocaine	Structure with comfort
Hyperdiluted Radiesse	CaHA	Skin tightening

QT® Fillers (South Korea)

QT® Fillers are a Korean hyaluronic acid (HA) dermal filler range developed to deliver reliable lifting capacity, smooth tissue integration, and clear product differentiation. Like many high-quality Korean fillers, QT focuses on high purity HA, consistent rheology, and cost-effective performance, making the range popular in markets where value, predictability, and versatility are important.

QT fillers are designed with a layered approach to facial rejuvenation, offering different gel strengths for superficial lines, mid-dermal correction, and deep structural support.

QT® Technology Explained

HCCL™ Cross-Linking Technology

(High Concentration Cross-Linked Hyaluronic Acid)

QT fillers are manufactured using HCCL™ technology, which creates a stable, cohesive HA gel network with controlled elasticity and lifting capacity.

Key Characteristics

- High-purity, non-animal HA

- Uniform gel consistency

- Good balance between firmness and spreadability

- Reliable shape retention

- Smooth extrusion and handling

Clinical Benefit: Predictable results with good longevity and controlled tissue integration.

Advanced Purification Process

- Low residual BDDE

- Reduced endotoxin levels

- Improved tolerability

Clinical Benefit: Lower inflammatory response and good safety profile when used appropriately.

The QT® Filler Range

Products, Technology & Indications

QT fillers are often grouped by depth and firmness, allowing straightforward product selection.

QT Hard

Technology: HCCL™

Indications

- Jawline definition
- Chin projection
- Structural facial contouring
- Deep supraperiosteal placement

Key Features

- Highest G' in the QT range
- Strong lifting and projection
- Excellent shape retention

Best for: Lower-face sculpting and foundational support.

QT Sub-Q

Technology: HCCL™

Indications

- Cheek volumisation
- Midface volume loss
- Facial contouring

Key Features

- High firmness
- Good lifting capacity

- Stable integration in deep planes

Best for: Deep volume restoration and facial framework.

QT Deep

Technology: HCCL™

Indications

- Nasolabial folds
- Marionette lines
- Moderate to deep wrinkles

Key Features

- Medium-high G'
- Balanced lift and flexibility

Best for: Classic wrinkle correction with support.

QT Soft

Technology: HCCL™

Indications

- Lips
- Perioral lines
- Superficial wrinkles

Key Features

- Softer gel texture
- Smooth spreadability
- Natural movement

Best for: Subtle lip enhancement and surface refinement.

QT Fine

Technology: HCCL™

Indications

- Fine lines
- Superficial wrinkles
- Tear troughs (experienced injectors only)

Key Features

- Low G'
- Minimal swelling profile
- Precise placement

Best for: Delicate areas and fine corrections.

QT Volume

Technology: HCCL™

Indications

- General volumisation
- Facial contouring
- Mild to moderate volume loss

Key Features

- Balanced firmness
- Versatile mid-to-deep placement

Best for: All-round volumisation where extreme firmness is not required

Clinical Considerations

- QT fillers use non-animal hyaluronic acid
- All QT fillers are reversible with hyaluronidase
- Clear firmness gradation assists safe product selection
- Suitable for:
    - Budget-conscious patients
    - Clinics seeking reliable, predictable fillers
    - Structured, stepwise facial rejuvenation

Summary Table

Product	Technology	Primary Use
QT Hard	HCCL	Jawline, chin, structure
QT Sub-Q	HCCL	Deep cheek volume
QT Deep	HCCL	Moderate–deep folds
QT Volume	HCCL	General volumisation
QT Soft	HCCL	Lips, superficial lines
QT Fine	HCCL	Fine lines, delicate areas

EPTQ® (Jetema Co. Ltd, South Korea)

EPTQ® is a premium Korean hyaluronic acid (HA) dermal filler range manufactured by Jetema, a globally recognised medical aesthetics company. EPTQ has gained strong international traction due to its high purity HA, advanced cross-linking technology, predictable rheology, and excellent value, while still meeting stringent global manufacturing standards.

The EPTQ range is designed to provide clear differentiation between lifting, contouring, and softer volumisation, making product selection intuitive for injectors and results consistent for patients.

EPTQ® Technology Explained

HET™ Technology

(High Elasticity Technology)

EPTQ fillers are produced using HET™ cross-linking, which creates a uniform, highly elastic gel structure with minimal residual BDDE.

Key Characteristics

- High purity HA
- Consistent particle size
- Strong elasticity with smooth extrusion
- Low endotoxin levels
- Excellent tissue integration

Clinical Benefit: Predictable lift, smooth placement, and reduced inflammatory response.

Low Residual BDDE Process

- Enhanced purification process
- Reduced risk of irritation and inflammation
- Improved safety profile

Clinical Benefit: Improved tolerability and suitability for a wide range of patients.

The EPTQ® Range

Products, Technology & Indications

EPTQ fillers are clearly categorised into Classic, S-Line, and E-Line, making selection based on firmness and indication straightforward.

EPTQ S 500

Technology: HET™

Indications

- Cheek augmentation
- Jawline contouring
- Chin projection
- Structural facial support

Key Features

- Highest G' in the EPTQ range
- Strong lifting and projection
- Excellent shape retention

Best for: Foundational structure and facial framework.

EPTQ S 300

Technology: HET™

Indications

- Midface volumisation
- Nasolabial folds
- Marionette lines

Key Features

- Balanced firmness and elasticity
- Smooth tissue integration

Best for: Moderate volume loss and contouring.

EPTQ S 100

Technology: HET™

Indications

- Fine lines
- Superficial wrinkles
- Tear troughs (experienced injectors only)

Key Features

- Lower G'
- Smooth spreadability
- Minimal swelling

Best for: Delicate areas and superficial corrections.

EPTQ E 400

Technology: HET™

Indications

- Cheek volume
- Facial contouring
- Structural support

Key Features

- Firm, cohesive gel

- High lifting power

Best for: Structural contouring with controlled projection.

EPTQ E 200

Technology: HET™

Indications

- Moderate wrinkles
- Nasolabial folds
- Marionette lines

Key Features

- Medium firmness
- Natural integration

Best for: Classic wrinkle correction.

EPTQ E 100

Technology: HET™

Indications

- Fine lines
- Superficial wrinkles
- Perioral lines

Key Features

- Soft gel consistency
- Smooth finish

Best for: Surface refinement and subtle correction.

EPTQ KISS

Technology: HET™

Indications

- Lip augmentation
- Lip contouring
- Lip hydration

Key Features

- Designed specifically for lips
- Soft, elastic texture
- Maintains natural lip movement

Best for: Natural-looking lip enhancement

EPTQ SENSE

Technology: HET™

Indications

- Skin hydration
- Texture improvement
- Fine lines

Key Features

- Skin booster rather than volumiser
- Micro-droplet technique
- Improves elasticity and glow

Best for: Skin rejuvenation without altering facial shape.

Clinical Considerations

- EPTQ fillers use non-animal HA

- High purity and low endotoxin levels

- All products are reversible with hyaluronidase

- Clear G' differentiation simplifies product choice

- Particularly popular where value, predictability, and versatility are important

Summary Table

Product	Technology	Primary Use
S 500	HET	Structural support
S 300	HET	Volume & contour
S 100	HET	Fine lines
E 400	HET	Contouring
E 200	HET	Moderate wrinkles
E 100	HET	Superficial lines
Kiss	HET	Lips
Sense	HET	Skin quality

HUGEL® (South Korea)

HUGEL® is a major South Korean pharmaceutical and medical aesthetics company with a rapidly expanding global footprint. While best known internationally for its neuromodulators, Hugel has also developed a high-quality hyaluronic acid (HA) dermal filler range, reflecting the Korean aesthetic philosophy of natural enhancement, smooth tissue integration, and skin quality preservation.

As Korean fillers gain increasing acceptance worldwide, Hugel represents a brand that is well positioned for current and future expansion into markets such as Australia, pending regulatory approvals.

HUGEL® Filler Technologies Explained

Advanced HA Cross-Linking & Purification Technology

Hugel fillers are manufactured using high-purity, non-animal hyaluronic acid, with a focus on:

- Uniform particle size
- Controlled cross-linking
- Low residual BDDE
- Low endotoxin levels

Key Characteristics

- Smooth, cohesive gel structure
- Good elasticity and lifting capacity
- Predictable handling and extrusion
- Reliable tissue integration

Clinical Benefit: Balanced performance across superficial, mid-dermal, and deep planes, with a focus on natural, harmonious results.

Korean Aesthetic Philosophy

Korean filler development traditionally prioritises:

- Soft tissue integration over exaggerated projection
- Skin hydration and quality alongside volume

- Gradual, natural-looking enhancement

Clinical Benefit: Fillers that are well suited to subtle contouring, refinement, and layered facial rejuvenation.

The HUGEL® Filler Range

Products, Technology & Indications

(Product naming and availability may vary by market)

HUGEL Volume

Technology: Cross-linked HA

Indications

- Cheek volumisation
- Midface volume loss
- Facial contouring

Key Features

- High G'
- Good lifting and projection
- Stable shape retention

Best for: Structural midface support and volume restoration.

HUGEL Deep

Technology: Cross-linked HA

Indications

- Nasolabial folds
- Marionette lines
- Moderate to deep wrinkles

Key Features

- Balanced firmness and elasticity
- Smooth integration in mid-dermal planes

Best for: Classic wrinkle correction with support.

HUGEL Fine

Technology: Cross-linked HA

Indications

- Fine lines
- Superficial wrinkles
- Perioral lines
- Tear troughs (experienced injectors only)

Key Features

- Low G'
- Smooth spreadability
- Minimal swelling profile

Best for: Delicate areas and surface refinement.

HUGEL Lips

Technology: Cross-linked HA

Indications

- Lip augmentation
- Lip definition
- Lip hydration

Key Features

- Soft, elastic gel
- Maintains natural lip movement
- Smooth finish

Best for: Natural, hydrated, expressive lips.

HUGEL Skin Booster

Technology: Lightly cross-linked HA

Indications

- Skin hydration
- Texture improvement
- Fine lines
- Dull or crepey skin

Key Features

- Micro-droplet technique
- Improves glow and elasticity
- Does not add volume

Best for: skin rejuvenation without altering facial shape.

Clinical Considerations

- Hugel fillers use non-animal hyaluronic acid
- Designed for smooth, controlled integration
- All HA fillers are reversible with hyaluronidase
- Product selection should consider:

o   Desired lift vs softness

o   Facial movement

o   Skin thickness

o   Cultural aesthetic preferences

Summary Table

Product	Technology	Primary Use
Hugel Volume	Cross-linked HA	Structural volume
Hugel Deep	Cross-linked HA	Moderate–deep folds
Hugel Fine	Cross-linked HA	Fine lines
Hugel Lips	Cross-linked HA	Lips
Hugel Skin Booster	Lightly cross-linked HA	Skin quality

Evolysse® (Evolus / Symatese)

Evolysse® is a next-generation hyaluronic acid (HA) filler line that represents one of the most recent technological advancements in the dermal filler category. Developed by Evolus in collaboration with Symatese, Evolysse uses an innovative Cold-X™ Technology manufacturing process to better preserve the natural structure of HA for smoother, more natural-looking results.

Unlike many traditional HA fillers made at higher temperatures, Cold-X™ technology processes HA at very low, near-freezing temperatures, which helps maintain longer HA chains and reduces the need for excessive cross-linking. This approach aims to produce a gel that integrates seamlessly into tissue, moves naturally with facial expressions, and may require less product for equivalent correction.

Evolysse® Technology Explained

Cold-X™ Technology

This proprietary manufacturing process is the defining feature of Evolysse fillers.

Key Advantages

- Preserves HA's natural structure: Low-temperature processing reduces fragmentation of the HA molecule.

- Natural tissue integration: The resulting gel integrates smoothly into facial tissue with minimal stiffness.

- Versatile performance: Designed to be injected at different levels depending on the area treated.

- Reduced hydrophilicity: Early clinical impressions suggest less unwanted swelling compared with some other HA fillers.

Clinical Benefit: Evolysse delivers a natural look and feel with effective correction of dynamic lines and facial volume loss, without the "overfilled" appearance that concerns many patients.

The Evolysse® Range

Products, Technology & Indications

As of 2025, the Evolysse line comprises two FDA-approved HA fillers, each formulated with Cold-X technology for specific treatment goals.

Evolysse Form

Technology: Cold-X™

Indications

- Moderate to deep smile lines and laugh lines (e.g., nasolabial folds)
- Facial contouring and volume restoration in deeper planes
- Structural support for areas requiring lift and definition

Key Features

- Firmer gel with cohesive structure
- Designed for deeper injection planes
- Provides lift as well as softening of folds

Best for: Patients needing substantial correction and support in deeper folds and facial contours.

Evolysse Smooth

Technology: Cold-X™

Indications

- Fine lines and superficial wrinkles
- Perioral lines
- Gentle contouring and refinement
- Subtle volume enhancement

Key Features

- Softer gel texture than Form
- Easier spreadability in more superficial planes
- Natural, subtle enhancement

Best for: Delicate areas such as around the mouth, mild folds, or early ageing signs where a softer touch is preferred.

Clinical Notes

- Both Evolysse Form and Evolysse Smooth are FDA-approved for correction of moderate-to-severe dynamic facial wrinkles and folds such as nasolabial folds in adults.

- Results typically last up to 12 months in many patients, though duration varies with treatment area, individual factors, and injector technique.

- Like other HA fillers, Evolysse gels are reversible with hyaluronidase if needed.

- The Cold-X™ process aims to minimize fragmentation and improve natural movement, potentially reducing the likelihood of stiffness or "puffy" results.

Summary Table

Product	Technology	Primary Use
Evolysse Form	Cold-X™	Deep volume, structural support, moderate–severe folds
Evolysse Smooth	Cold-X™	Superficial lines, fine wrinkle refinement, subtle enhancement.

STYLAGE® (Vivacy Laboratories, France)

STYLAGE® is a premium French hyaluronic acid (HA) dermal filler range developed by Laboratoires Vivacy. The brand is well known for integrating antioxidant technology into its fillers, positioning Stylage not only as a volumising and contouring solution, but also as a product range designed to protect skin from oxidative stress and premature ageing.

Stylage fillers are recognised for their smooth texture, versatility, and refined aesthetic outcomes, making them suitable for both structural work and delicate, superficial corrections.

Stylage® Technologies Explained

IPN-Like® Technology

(InterPenetrated Network-Like Technology)

Stylage fillers are manufactured using IPN-Like cross-linking, which creates a three-dimensional HA network that balances firmness with flexibility.

Key Characteristics

- Strong gel cohesion
- Smooth tissue integration
- Good elasticity
- Controlled projection and spread

Clinical Benefit: Predictable lift with natural facial movement and good longevity.

Antioxidant Enrichment (Mannitol or Sorbitol)

A defining feature of Stylage is the inclusion of antioxidants within many products.

Why this matters

- Antioxidants help reduce oxidative degradation of HA
- May prolong filler longevity
- Can reduce post-injection inflammation and swelling

Clinical Benefit: Improved tolerance, smoother healing, and enhanced durability of results.

The STYLAGE® Range

Products, Technology & Indications

Stylage fillers are grouped clearly by depth, firmness, and indication, making selection intuitive.

Stylage XXL

Technology: IPN-Like + Mannitol

Indications

- Cheek volumisation
- Jawline contouring
- Chin projection
- Structural facial support

Key Features

- Very high G'
- Strong lifting and projection
- Excellent shape retention

Best for: Deep structural support and facial framework.

Stylage XL

Technology: IPN-Like + Mannitol

Indications

- Midface volume restoration
- Facial contouring
- Deep nasolabial folds

Key Features

- High firmness

- Smooth integration

Best for: Volume restoration with contour control.

Stylage L

Technology: IPN-Like + Mannitol

Indications

- Moderate to deep wrinkles
- Nasolabial folds
- Marionette lines

Key Features

- Balanced lift and flexibility
- Good longevity

Best for: Classic wrinkle correction with support.

Stylage M

Technology: IPN-Like + Mannitol

Indications

- Moderate wrinkles
- Perioral lines
- Facial refinement

Key Features

- Medium G'
- Natural movement

Best for: Dynamic areas requiring softness with support.

Stylage S

Technology: IPN-Like + Sorbitol

Indications

- Fine lines
- Superficial wrinkles
- Perioral lines

Key Features

- Soft gel consistency
- Precise placement
- Minimal swelling

Best for: Surface refinement and fine line correction.

Stylage Special Lips®

Technology: IPN-Like + Mannitol

Indications

- Lip augmentation
- Lip contouring
- Lip hydration

Key Features

- Designed specifically for lips
- Soft, flexible texture
- Maintains natural lip movement

Best for: Natural, expressive lip enhancement.

Stylage Hydro® / HydroMax®

Technology: IPN-Like + Sorbitol

Indications

- Skin hydration

- Texture improvement

- Fine lines

- Crepey skin

Key Features

- Skin booster, not a volumiser

- Improves elasticity and glow

- HydroMax offers enhanced hydration and longevity

Best for: Skin quality improvement without volume change.

Clinical Considerations

- Stylage fillers use non-animal HA

- Many products include lidocaine for comfort

- Antioxidant content may reduce swelling and HA breakdown

- All Stylage fillers are reversible with hyaluronidase

- Suitable for:

  o Patients prone to swelling

  o Refinement and natural aesthetics

  o Structured yet flexible facial rejuvenation

Summary Table

Product	Technology	Primary Use
XXL	IPN-Like + Mannitol	Structural volume
XL	IPN-Like + Mannitol	Deep volume
L	IPN-Like + Mannitol	Deep wrinkles
M	IPN-Like + Mannitol	Moderate wrinkles
S	IPN-Like + Sorbitol	Fine lines
Special Lips	IPN-Like + Mannitol	Lips
Hydro / HydroMax	IPN-Like + Sorbitol	Skin quality

CHROMA® (Croma-Pharma GmbH, Austria)

CHROMA® is an Austrian pharmaceutical company with a strong European reputation for medical-grade injectables, including hyaluronic acid (HA) dermal fillers, skin boosters, and regenerative products. Croma is particularly known for its strict manufacturing standards, pharmaceutical-level purity, and safety-first design philosophy.

CHROMA fillers are developed to provide predictable rheology, smooth tissue integration, and a broad portfolio that allows injectors to treat everything from delicate superficial lines to deep structural volume.

CHROMA® Technologies Explained

Monophasic Cross-Linked HA Technology

CHROMA fillers are produced as homogeneous monophasic gels, meaning the HA particles are evenly distributed throughout the gel.

Key Characteristics

- Smooth, cohesive consistency

- Uniform extrusion force

- Reduced lumpiness and palpability

- Predictable tissue behaviour

Clinical Benefit: Even integration into tissue with controlled spread and reliable aesthetic outcomes.

High-Purity Manufacturing Standards

- Non-animal sourced hyaluronic acid

- Low residual BDDE

- Low endotoxin levels

- Pharmaceutical-grade quality control

Clinical Benefit: Excellent tolerability and safety profile, particularly important in delicate facial areas.

The CHROMA® Filler Range
Products, Technology & Indications
(Product names may vary slightly by market)

CHROMA Volume
Technology: Monophasic cross-linked HA
Indications

- Cheek volumisation

- Midface volume loss

- Facial contouring

- Structural support
Key Features

- High G'

- Strong lifting and projection

- Stable shape retention
Best for: Foundational volume and facial framework.

CHROMA Deep
Technology: Monophasic cross-linked HA
Indications

- Nasolabial folds

- Marionette lines

- Moderate to deep wrinkles
Key Features

- Balanced firmness and elasticity

- Smooth mid-dermal integration
Best for: Classic wrinkle correction with support.

CHROMA Derm
Technology: Monophasic cross-linked HA
Indications

- Moderate wrinkles

- Facial refinement

- Dynamic areas requiring flexibility
Key Features

- Medium G'

• Natural movement
Best for: Areas where expression needs to be preserved.

CHROMA Fine
Technology: Monophasic cross-linked HA
Indications

• Fine lines

• Superficial wrinkles

• Perioral lines

• Tear troughs *(experienced injectors only)*
Key Features

• Low G'

• Smooth spreadability

• Minimal swelling profile
Best for: Delicate areas and fine corrections.

CHROMA Lips
Technology: Monophasic cross-linked HA

Indications

• Lip augmentation

• Lip definition

• Lip hydration
Key Features

• Soft, elastic gel

• Maintains natural lip movement

• Smooth finish
Best for: Natural-looking, hydrated lips.

CHROMA Skin Booster

Technology: Lightly cross-linked HA
Indications

- Skin hydration

- Texture improvement

- Fine lines

- Dull or crepey skin
Key Features

- Micro-droplet technique

- Improves elasticity and glow

- No volumisation
Best for: Skin rejuvenation without changing facial shape.

Clinical Considerations

- CHROMA fillers are HA-based and reversible with hyaluronidase

- Designed for smooth, predictable integration

- Suitable for:

  - Refinement and natural aesthetics

  - Layered facial rejuvenation

  - Patients prioritising safety and tolerance

Fillmed — A Scientific Aesthetic Medicine Brand

Laboratoires FILLMED is a French aesthetic medicine company founded in 1978 by Dr. Michel Tordjman, a pioneer in combining clinical science with anti-ageing treatments for dermatologists, plastic surgeons and trained aesthetic medicine professionals. The brand has a long track record in developing medical-grade solutions for skin rejuvenation, tissue quality improvement and age-related volume loss.

Fillmed products are designed to correct signs of ageing, revitalise skin and enhance facial structure, using biocompatible hyaluronic acid and advanced formulations. The company's portfolio spans injectable fillers, mesotherapy solutions, peels and professional skin-quality boosters — all aimed at delivering reliable, natural-looking results backed by science.

Core Philosophy & Technology

Tri-Hyal® Technology

A hallmark of Fillmed's dermal fillers, Tri-Hyal® technology combines three different molecular weights of hyaluronic acid (free, long chains and very long chains) in a balanced formula. This enables gradual integration into tissue, better hydration, improved elasticity, and a smoother, more natural outcome compared with single-weight HA fillers.

Non-Animal Hyaluronic Acid

Fillmed's products are made of non-animal origin HA, reducing the risk of allergic reactions and improving biocompatibility — a standard in modern medical aesthetics.

The Art Filler Range — Dermal Fillers for Different Aesthetic Goals

Fillmed's Art Filler® collection is its flagship range of injectable dermal fillers, each tailored to specific treatment needs within facial rejuvenation:

1. Art Filler Fine Lines

- Target: Superficial or fine wrinkles (e.g., around eyes, mouth and forehead).

- Profile: Softer, smoother gel designed for delicate areas.

- Benefits: Subtle wrinkle smoothing with natural integration.

- With Lidocaine: Often includes a small percentage of lidocaine to improve comfort during injection.

2. Art Filler Universal

- Target: Versatile, medium-to-deep wrinkles and general facial contouring.

- Use: Can be used for smoothing folds (e.g., nasolabial lines), restoring mid-facial volume and light lip contouring.

- Composition: Balanced level of HA with lidocaine for comfort and hydration.

- Notes: A go-to filler when a practitioner wants one product that performs well in multiple areas of the face.

3. Art Filler Volume

- Target: Deep volume restoration — cheeks, chin, jawline and temples.

- Profile: Higher cohesivity and cross-linking to support deeper tissue structure and volume replacement.

- Benefits: Adds lift and shape to areas with age-related volume loss.

4. Art Filler Lips & Lips Soft

- Art Filler Lips: Designed for more pronounced lip volume and projection.

- Art Filler Lips Soft: A gentler formulation for natural lip enhancement, contour and hydration.

- Both include Lidocaine: For greater comfort during lip injections.

- Indications: Lip augmentation, border definition, smoothing perioral lines.

Other Hyaluronic Acid-Based Solutions

Beyond the classic Art Filler line, Fillmed also offers HA-based mesotherapy and hydration boosters such as:

M-HA 10

- A pure, non-crosslinked hyaluronic acid solution used in mesotherapy to replenish hydration, improve skin tone and elasticity, and soften fine lines.

- Ideal for superficial rejuvenation on areas like face, neck, décolletage and hands.

How Fillmed Fits Into the Aesthetic Medicine Landscape

Fillmed stands out for:

- Its medical-science foundation and long heritage since the late 1970s.

- The Tri-Hyal® approach that emphasises skin biology and tissue integration.

- A broad range that spans fine lines, volume replacement and skin hydration, giving practitioners flexibility across treatment plans.

Summary : Filler Brands and Their Ranges

Dermal fillers are not interchangeable products. Each brand and range has been developed with specific technologies, gel properties, and clinical purposes in mind. Understanding these differences is essential for achieving safe, natural, and long-lasting results.

This chapter has explored the major global filler brands — European, Korean, American, and emerging technologies —

highlighting how rheology, cross-linking, and formulation influence how a filler behaves in the face.

Key Points for Patients

1. One Face, Many Filler Types

There is no single "best filler." Different areas of the face require fillers that:

- Lift and support (cheeks, jawline, chin)
- Move naturally (smile lines, lips)
- Blend seamlessly (under-eyes, fine lines)
- Improve skin quality (hydration, elasticity)

Your injector chooses the filler based on your anatomy and goals, not brand popularity.

2. Technology Matters

Fillers differ in:

- Firmness (G')
- Flexibility and stretch
- Water attraction and swelling potential
- Longevity
- How they integrate into tissue

These differences determine whether a filler lifts, softens, hydrates, or stimulates collagen.

3. Natural Results Are Designed, Not Injected

The most natural outcomes come from:

- Using the correct filler in the correct layer

- Restoring structure rather than overfilling

- Respecting facial movement and proportions

Good filler work should enhance how you already look — not change who you are.

4. Safety Comes Before Aesthetics

All dermal fillers are medical devices. Safe treatment depends on:

- Injector training and anatomical knowledge

- Appropriate product selection

- Conservative dosing

- Understanding reversibility and risk zones

Choosing an experienced injector is more important than choosing a brand.

5. Longevity Is Individual

How long fillers last varies depending on:

- Product type

- Area treated

- Facial movement

- Individual metabolism

Longer-lasting is not always better — adjustability and safety are key.

Key Points for Injectors

1. Brand Ranges Exist for a Reason

Each filler range offers:

- A spectrum of firmness and elasticity

- Products designed for different facial depths

- Specific behaviour in static vs dynamic areas

Mastering a range allows precision, predictability, and layered treatment planning.

2. Choose Fillers Based on Tissue, Not Habit

Clinical decision-making should be guided by:

- Skin thickness

- Degree of volume loss

- Movement patterns

- Treatment depth

- Patient age and hormonal status

Different tissues require different gel behaviours.

3. Reversibility and Risk Management Are Core Skills

- HA fillers allow reversibility and flexibility

- Non-HA fillers require advanced training

- Product choice must reflect injector experience and patient risk profile

Safety planning is part of artistry.

4. Modern Aesthetics Go Beyond Volume

Today's best outcomes combine:

- Structural HA fillers

- Flexible fillers for movement

- Skin boosters

- Biostimulators for collagen support

A multimodal approach delivers long-term facial health, not just short-term correction.

5. Confidence Comes from Understanding

Injectors who understand:

- Filler technologies
- Rheology
- Brand differences
- Anatomical application

achieve better results with less product and fewer complications.

Dermal fillers are tools — not trends.

The success of any treatment depends on:

- The right filler
- In the right place
- At the right depth
- For the right patient
- Used by the right injector

When filler brands and ranges are understood and respected, outcomes become natural, safe, and sustainable.

CHAPTER 31: FILLER MIGRATION: CAUSES, ANATOMY, PREVENTION, AND SOLUTIONS

What Is Filler Migration?

Filler migration occurs when dermal filler moves from the intended injection site to an adjacent or unintended area. This can cause aesthetic concerns (such as uneven swelling, puffiness, or unnatural contours) and, in some cases, functional issues (like obstructed lymphatic drainage under the eyes).

While migration can happen with any type of filler, it is most commonly seen with hyaluronic acid (HA) fillers, which are more mobile compared to thicker, more cohesive fillers like calcium hydroxyapatite (Radiesse) or poly-L-lactic acid (Sculptra).

Why Does Filler Migration Happen?

Filler migration can occur due to several anatomical, injection technique, and product-related factors:

1. Incorrect Placement in High-Movement Areas

Fillers injected into areas that experience frequent movement (e.g., lips, perioral region, under-eyes) are more likely to disperse over time.

The orbicularis oris (around the mouth) and orbicularis oculi (around the eyes) are constantly contracting, which can cause fillers to move or spread.

2. Poor Injection Depth

Superficial injection (too close to the skin surface) can allow the filler to move more easily compared to deep injections placed near the periosteum (bone layer).

Example: If cheek filler is injected too close to the surface, it may drift downward into the lower face due to gravity and facial movement.

3. Overfilling or Overcorrection

Injecting excessive filler into one area increases the risk of it spreading beyond the intended site.

This is particularly problematic in the lips, where an overfilled vermillion border can lead to the duck lip effect or migration into the white roll of the lip.

4. Soft Gel-Like Fillers

Softer, less crosslinked fillers (e.g., those used for lip augmentation or tear troughs) have a higher tendency to migrate compared to more structured, cohesive fillers used for deep structural support.

Some filler brands, such as those using Vycross technology (e.g., Juvederm Volbella, Volift, Voluma), may integrate well but can also be more prone to migration over time.

5. Muscle Activity & Gravity

Frequent muscle movement (e.g., talking, chewing, smiling) can push filler away from the intended site.

Gravity plays a role in downward migration, particularly in areas like the temples and cheeks, where misplaced filler can drift lower.

6. Lymphatic Blockage & Fluid Retention

The under-eye region is particularly prone to filler migration because the lymphatic drainage system is delicate.

If filler is injected too superficially or too close to lymphatic channels, it can trap fluid, leading to chronic puffiness or festoon-like swelling.

7. Repeated Treatments Without Full Dissolution

Over time, multiple layers of filler build up, creating an unnatural, doughy appearance.

Filler that was not fully dissolved from previous treatments may continue migrating even after new injections.

Where Does Filler Migrate?

1. Temple Filler Moving to the Cheek

If temple filler is injected too superficially, it can drift downward into the cheek over time.

This occurs because the temporalis muscle and fascia are connected to the zygomatic (cheek) region, allowing movement between these compartments.

2. Under-Eye Filler Causing Puffy Eyes

When filler is placed too superficially in the tear trough, it can obstruct lymphatic drainage, leading to persistent swelling and fluid retention.

This is often seen when soft fillers (like Volbella or Belotero Balance) are placed in the wrong tissue plane.

3. Lip Filler Spreading Beyond the Lip Border

Overfilled lips may push filler beyond the vermillion border, causing a duck lip or filler Mustache appearance.

This often occurs when filler is injected too superficially or in excessive amounts, leading to migration into the white roll or perioral area.

4. Nasolabial Fold Filler Spreading Laterally

Fillers injected into the nasolabial folds (smile lines) can sometimes spread outward, creating a bloated or widened appearance.

This is due to poor injection technique or placing filler too superficially.

5. Jawline Filler Moving Into the Neck

If too much filler is injected too low on the jawline, it may spread into the submental (under-chin) area, leading to an unnatural fullness or heaviness in the lower face.

How to Prevent Filler Migration

1. Proper Injection Techniques

Deep injections (near bone or deeper fat compartments) reduce movement.

Avoid overfilling in soft areas (e.g., lips, tear troughs).

Use microbolus techniques-small, precise amounts instead of large boluses.

Cannula technique may help reduce migration compared to needles in certain areas.

2. Choosing the Right Filler for the Right Area

Higher G (stiff, cohesive fillers) for structural support (e.g., cheeks, jawline).

Lower G (soft, fluid fillers) for mobile areas (e.g., lips, tear troughs).

Avoid highly crosslinked, dense fillers in delicate areas (e.g., under-eyes).

3. Spacing Out Treatments

Avoid layering too much filler over old injections.

Consider hyaluronidase (filler dissolver) before re-treating a migrated area.

Solutions for Filler Migration: Hyaluronidase

If filler migration occurs, it can often be corrected using hyaluronidase, an enzyme that breaks down hyaluronic acid-based fillers.

How Hyaluronidase Works

Hyaluronidase is a naturally occurring enzyme that dissolves HA fillers within hours to days.

It can be injected in small, targeted doses to selectively remove migrated or misplaced filler.

The effects are immediate but may take up to 48 hours for full results.

In some cases, a second or third session may be needed if the filler is deeply embedded.

When to Use Hyaluronidase

Under-eye puffiness caused by migrated filler.

Lip filler that has spread beyond the lip border.

Temple or cheek filler that has drifted into unwanted areas.

Overfilled, lumpy, or asymmetrical filler placements.

Can All Fillers Be Dissolved?

Hyaluronic acid fillers (e.g., Juvederm, Restylane, Belotero, Teoxane) can be dissolved.

Non-HA fillers (e.g., Radiesse, Sculptra, Bellafill) CANNOT be dissolved and may require alternative treatments like surgical removal.

Conclusion

Filler migration is caused by poor injection technique, overfilling, anatomical movement, and soft gel-like fillers in high-motion areas.

Common migration sites include under-eyes (causing puffiness), lips (spreading beyond the vermillion border), and cheeks (dropping from the temple).

Prevention strategies include using the correct filler type, proper injection depth, and avoiding excessive product placement.

Hyaluronidase is the go-to solution for dissolving migrated hyaluronic acid fillers.

Choosing an experienced injector who understands anatomy and rheology is critical to avoiding filler migration.

When considering the use of Hyalase (hyaluronidase) in individuals with known bee or wasp sting allergies, caution is imperative due to potential cross-reactivity. Hyaluronidase is an enzyme present in both bee and wasp venoms, facilitating the spread of venom through tissues. This structural similarity can lead to the immune system recognizing medical hyaluronidase as a foreign substance, potentially triggering allergic reactions ranging from mild skin irritation to severe anaphylaxis. Cross-reactivity occurs when the immune system identifies structurally similar proteins from different sources as the same allergen. In this context, the hyaluronidase enzyme in insect venom shares epitopes with medical hyaluronidase, leading to potential cross-reactive allergic responses. Clinical Implications:

•**Risk Assessment**: Before administering hyaluronidase, it's crucial to assess patients for a history of severe reactions to bee or wasp stings.

CHAPTER 32: BRUISING & COSMETIC PROCEDURES: WHAT TO EXPECT & HOW TO MANAGE IT

Bruising is a common side effect after injectable treatments, especially in delicate areas like the lips, under-eyes, and forehead. While not everyone bruises, certain factors increase the risk. Here's how to minimize, treat, and camouflage bruises effectively.

Am I Going to Bruise?

Risk Factors for Bruising:

• Thin or fragile skin (more common in mature skin)

• Use of blood thinners (aspirin, ibuprofen, fish oil, alcohol, etc.)

• History of easy bruising or bleeding disorders

• Highly vascular areas (e.g., lips and under-eyes)

• Aggressive injection technique (needle vs. cannula)

If you're prone to bruising, let your injector know beforehand!

What to Stop Using Before Treatment (Prevention Tips)

Avoid These for at Least 5-7 Days Before Treatment:

• Blood Thinners & NSAIDs (Aspirin, Ibuprofen, Naproxen)

- Alcohol (Increases blood vessel dilation)

- Omega-3 Supplements (Fish oil, flaxseed oil)

- Vitamin E & Herbal Supplements (Ginkgo, Garlic, Ginseng, St. John's Wort)

- Caffeine (Reduces platelet function)

Consider Taking Before Treatment:

- Arnica Tablets or Gel – Helps minimize bruising & swelling

- Bromelain (Pineapple Enzyme) – Anti-inflammatory properties

How to Prevent Bruising on the Day of Treatment

Hydrate well & eat before your appointment (to stabilize blood sugar)

Avoid strenuous exercise before & after

Apply ice packs immediately post-treatment

Use a cannula where possible (less trauma to blood vessels)

How to Treat Bruises (Post-Treatment Care)

First 24 Hours:

- Cold Compress (10 min on, 10 min off) – Reduces swelling & bleeding under the skin

- Avoid touching or massaging the area (unless instructed)

- Keep your head elevated (reduces blood pooling)

After 48 Hours:

- Warm Compresses – Improves circulation & speeds up healing

- Arnica Gel or Cream – Apply directly to bruised areas

- Bromelain Supplements – Continue to help with inflammation

- Vitamin K Cream – Strengthens capillaries & fades bruises

How to Camouflage a Bruise with Makeup

Step-by-Step Concealing Process:

Apply Lipstick/Color Corrector First

- For Purple/Blue Bruises: Use red or orange-toned lipstick

- For Green/Yellow Bruises: Use peach or salmon tones

Set with Translucent Powder

- Prevents smudging & ensures longevity

Apply Full-Coverage Concealer/Foundation

- Use a thick, high-pigment concealer like Dermablend or Kryolan

Final Setting Powder or Spray

- Camouflage powder locks in coverage for the day

Iron Staining (Hemosiderin Staining) from Bruising Around the Eyes: Causes & Treatment

Iron staining, also known as hemosiderin staining, occurs when red blood cells break down after a bruise, leaving iron deposits in the skin. This can result in persistent yellow-brown or grayish discoloration, particularly around the under-eyes, where the skin is thin and prone to pigmentation issues.

Why Does Iron Staining Happen?

Occurs when blood leaks into tissues from damaged capillaries

Hemosiderin (iron-containing pigment) is left behind as the body breaks down the bruise

More common in individuals with fair or thin skin

Can be prolonged if poor circulation slows clearance

How to Treat Iron Staining Around the Eyes

Key Approach: Break down iron deposits, improve circulation, and speed up cell turnover.

Topical Treatments to Fade Staining

Vitamin C Serum – Antioxidant properties help brighten the skin and reduce discoloration (e.g., Skinceuticals C E Ferulic, Medik8 C-Tetra).

Iron-Chelating Creams (Lactoferrin or EDTA-based) – Help remove iron buildup in the skin (e.g., iS Clinical C Eye Serum, Dermaceutic Mela Cream).

Retinol (Vitamin A) or Peptides – Stimulates collagen renewal and fades pigmentation (e.g., Medik8 Crystal Retinal, SkinCeuticals A.G.E. Eye Complex).

Arnica & Bromelain Creams – Reduce inflammation & improve circulation (e.g., Arnicare Gel, Auriderm XO Cream).

AMERIGEL Care Lotion with Oakin® (oak extract) has been shown to help resolve Hemosiderin Staining through its unique formulation. The Care Lotion's fast absorbing formulation penetrates through the outer layers of skin allowing the oak extract to bond with the accumulated Iron deposits, helping the body to break down and naturally reabsorb the smaller iron particles. This process continues with every application of AMERIGEL Care Lotion until the deposits have been fully dissolved.

In-Clinic Treatments for Faster Results

Q-Switched or Picosecond Laser – Targets hemosiderin pigment directly to break it down.

Chemical Peels (Low Strength TCA, Mandelic, or Lactic Acid) – Speeds up skin cell turnover and fades staining.

Microneedling with PRP or Vitamin C Infusion – Stimulates collagen remodeling and reduces stubborn pigmentation.

At-Home Skincare Routine for Long-Term Improvement

Daily SPF 50+ (Essential!) – Prevents further pigmentation (e.g., ISDIN Eryfotona Ageless, EltaMD UV Clear).

Hydration & Lymphatic Drainage Massage – Improves circulation, reducing stagnant pigmentation.

Healthy Diet (Iron-Rich Foods + Vitamin C) – Supports blood vessel health & skin regeneration.

How Long Does Iron Staining Last?

Mild cases: Fades within a few weeks with proper skincare.

Moderate cases: Can persist for months without intervention.

Severe cases: May require laser or professional treatments to fully resolve.

Final Thoughts

Iron staining after bruising is stubborn but treatable.

Early intervention with Vitamin C, retinol, and gentle exfoliation helps speed up recovery.

If discoloration persists beyond 3 months, consider laser or peels for faster resolution.

CHAPTER 33: BIO-STIMULANTS: HOW THEY WORK & WHY THEY'RE GAME-CHANGERS IN AESTHETIC MEDICINE

What Are Bio-Stimulants?

Bio-stimulants are injectable treatments that stimulate the body's natural collagen production rather than simply adding volume like traditional hyaluronic acid (HA) fillers. They work by triggering a wound-healing response, leading to gradual and long-lasting skin rejuvenation and structural support.

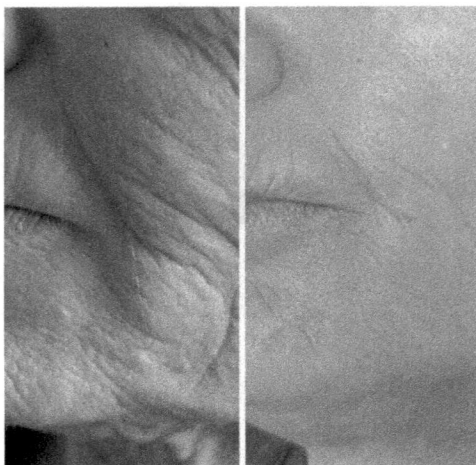

Two of the most well-known bio-stimulants in aesthetic medicine are Sculptra (poly-L-lactic acid) and Radiesse (calcium hydroxylapatite, CaHA).

How Do Sculptra & Radiesse Work?

Bio-Stimulant	Primary Component	Mechanism of Action	Collagen Type Stimulated
Sculptra	Poly-L-lactic acid (PLLA)	Stimulates fibroblasts to increase collagen production over time	Primarily Type I Collagen (strong structural collagen)
Radiesse	Calcium hydroxylapatite (CaHA) microspheres	Provides immediate volume while stimulating fibroblasts for long-term collagen production	Primarily Type I & Type III Collagen (Type III is found in youthful skin)

Sculptra (PLLA) Long-Lasting, Natural Rejuvenation

Works gradually by stimulating fibroblasts to produce Type I collagen, which supports the skin's structure and firmness.

Results appear over 3-6 months after a series of three sessions, spaced one month apart.

Lasts up to two years, but annual maintenance is recommended due to ongoing fat and bone volume loss (especially for patients on weight loss medications like Ozempic).

Injectors can target deeper layers even down to the bone for profound rejuvenation.

Radiesse (CaHA) Instant & Long-Term Lifting Power

Provides immediate volume due to its thick, opaque gel carrier, making it ideal for hand rejuvenation and deep facial volumization.

Over time, stimulates both Type I and Type III collagen, enhancing skin elasticity and firmness.

Can be used undiluted for deep structural support (cheeks, jawline) or hyperdiluted for skin rejuvenation (decolletage, neck, arms, abdomen).

Indications for Use: Where Do Bio-Stimulants Work Best?

Sculptra :Best for Gradual, Natural Full-Face Rejuvenation

Cheeks, temples, jawline (treats deeper fat and bone loss).

Pre-jowl sulcus & marionette lines (restores structural integrity).

Decolletage arms, knees (firms and thickens aging skin).

Buttocks and hip dips (for non-surgical body contouring).

Radiesse Best for Instant Lift & Targeted Rejuvenation

Hands (its opacity hides vein prominence and volume loss).

Jawline and chin (provides immediate contouring).

Hyperdiluted for skin rejuvenation on neck, arms, thighs, and abdomen.

Hyperdiluted Sculptra & Radiesse for Skin Rejuvenation

Hyperdiluted versions of Sculptra and Radiesse are fantastic for improving skin quality, texture, and elasticity.

When diluted with saline and lidocaine, they can be injected more superficially to treat crepey, sagging skin.

Best for neck, décolletage, arms, and knees, where traditional fillers may not be suitable.

Why Sculptra Is My Favorite Bio-Stimulant (After PRP)

Sculptra provides gradual, natural volume restoration , patients look like a better version of themselves, not overfilled.

It's a long-term collagen stimulator, meaning the results continue improving over time.

The ability to target deep fat pads and bone allows for profound facial rejuvenation.

 A must-have treatment for patients experiencing facial volume loss due to aging or weight loss (e.g., Ozempic users).

Conclusion: Bio-Stimulants Are the Future of Aesthetic Medicine

Sculptra (PLLA) and Radiesse (CaHA) stimulate collagen for long-term rejuvenation.

Sculptra boosts Type I collagen, while Radiesse enhances both Type I and Type III collagen.

Treatment areas include the face, hands, neck, and even body contouring (buttocks, arms, knees).

Hyperdiluted versions improve skin laxity and texture without adding bulk.

For optimal results, patients should complete a series of treatments and maintain yearly top-ups.

With bio-stimulants, we are shifting from simply filling lines to rebuilding the skin's foundation, allowing for natural, long-lasting rejuvenation.

Profhilo® Structura: Advanced Facial Rejuvenation

Profhilo® Structura is an innovative injectable treatment developed to address deeper structural changes in the face associated with aging. Building upon the original Profhilo® formulation, Structura focuses on regenerating and repositioning superficial facial fat layers to enhance facial contours and provide a natural lifting effect.

Composition and Technology

Utilizing the patented NAHYCO® technology, Profhilo® Structura combines 45 mg of high molecular weight hyaluronic acid (H-HA) with 45 mg of low molecular weight hyaluronic acid (L-HA) per 2 mL syringe. This thermal stabilization process creates hybrid cooperative complexes (HCC) without the need for chemical cross-linking agents, resulting in a purer and more biocompatible product.

Mechanism of Action

Injected into the superficial fat compartments of the face, particularly the preauricular area, Profhilo® Structura stimulates the regeneration of adipose tissue. This process counteracts age-related fat loss and tissue descent, effectively restoring facial volume and contour. The treatment promotes collagen production and enhances skin firmness, leading to a rejuvenated and lifted appearance.

Treatment Protocol

The recommended protocol involves two treatment sessions spaced one month apart. Each session consists of injecting 1 mL of Profhilo® Structura into each side of the face using a 25G x 50 mm cannula, targeting the superficial fat compartments. Clinical studies have demonstrated significant improvements in facial volume and wrinkle reduction, with results maintained for at least three months post-treatment.

Distinction from Original Profhilo®

While both Profhilo® and Profhilo® Structura utilize hyaluronic acid-based formulations, they serve different purposes:

• **Profhilo®:** Primarily enhances skin hydration and elasticity by stimulating collagen and elastin production in the dermis, without adding volume.

• **Profhilo® Structura**: Targets deeper layers to restore facial fat compartments, providing structural support and a lifting effect, thereby addressing more pronounced signs of aging.

In summary, Profhilo® Structura offers a novel approach to facial rejuvenation by focusing on the restoration of subcutaneous fat and structural support, delivering natural-looking results for individuals experiencing age-related facial volume loss and sagging.

Profhilo Structura: for Sinkers & Saggers.

Unlike regular Profhilo, which uses the BAP (Bio Aesthetic Points) technique with needle injections, Profhilo Structura is administered exclusively with a cannula, allowing for better diffusion, reduced trauma, and targeted tissue support.

Profhilo Structura

Sinkers

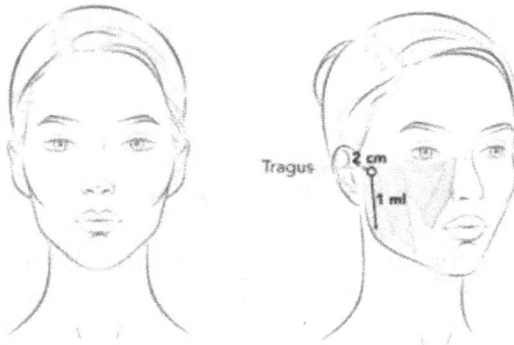

Saggers

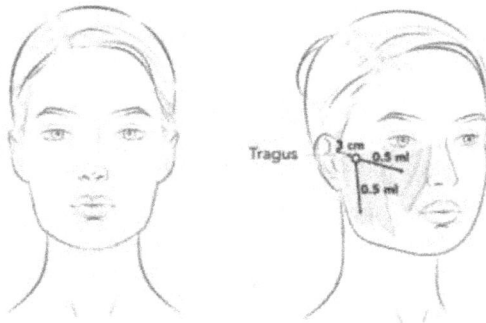

Sinkers vs. Saggers: Understanding the Two Aging Patterns

1. Sinkers – Individuals who lose volume due to fat pad depletion, bone resorption, and skin thinning.

• Common Areas: Midface, temples, preauricular region, jawline

• Treatment Goal: Restore support and prevent further structural collapse

2. Saggers – Individuals with skin laxity and tissue descent, causing jowling, deep marionette lines, and lower face drooping.

• Common Areas: Jawline, submalar (SUMO) region, neck

• Treatment Goal: Tighten and lift skin by enhancing collagen and elastin production

Injection Techniques for Profhilo Structura: Sinkers vs. Saggers
1. Injection Technique for Sinkers (Structural Loss & Volume Depletion)

Cannula: 22G

Entry Point: Preauricular (near the ear)

Injection Plane: Deep subcutaneous layer (above SMAS)

Technique:

• Retrograde threading – Injecting product while withdrawing the cannula, ensuring even distribution

• Targeting deep fat compartments for improved facial support

Goal:

• Reinforce structural integrity of volume-depleted areas

• Improve hydration and skin quality

• Prevent further sinking of facial tissues

2. Injection Technique for Saggers (Skin Laxity & Drooping)

Cannula: 25G

Entry Points:

• SUMO area (submalar fat pad) – To support midface tissue

• Preauricular (near the ear) – To tighten jawline and reduce jowling

Injection Plane: Superficial subcutaneous layer

Technique:

• Soft fanning technique – Spreading the product evenly across legs zygmatic bone and pre auricular (lateral cheek) .

• Emphasis on collagen stimulation rather than volume replacement

Goal:

• Strengthen skin support structures

• Enhance elasticity and skin density

• Reduce sagging and improve skin texture

Why Use a Cannula for Profhilo Structura?

• **Safer Delivery** – Reduces risk of vascular compromise

• **Less Bruising & Swelling** – Fewer entry points compared to multiple needle injections

• **Better Product Diffusion** – Spreads smoothly across treatment zones for natural integration.

GOURI

GOURI is an innovative, fully liquid polycaprolactone (PCL) injectable developed to stimulate natural collagen production, offering comprehensive skin rejuvenation. Unlike traditional fillers that primarily add volume, GOURI enhances the skin's structural integrity by promoting collagen synthesis, leading to improved elasticity and a more youthful appearance.

Key Features of GOURI:

• **Composition**: GOURI utilizes 100% liquid PCL, a biodegradable and biocompatible polymer, ensuring a natural integration into the skin.

• **Mechanism of Action**: Upon injection, GOURI spreads evenly across the treatment area, stimulating fibroblasts to produce collagen. This process gradually restores skin elasticity and firmness, addressing signs of aging such as fine lines and wrinkles.

• **Treatment Areas**: GOURI is versatile and can be used on various facial regions, including the cheeks, nasolabial folds, and areas with noticeable sagging or loss of elasticity.

• **Procedure**: The treatment involves injecting GOURI into specific points of the face using either a 5-point injection technique or a cannula method. The choice of technique depends on the patient's needs and the practitioner's assessment.

• **Results and Longevity**: Patients may begin to notice improvements within a few weeks post-treatment, with optimal results typically observed after multiple sessions. The effects of GOURI can last between 6 to 12 months, depending on individual factors and the treatment plan.

Benefits of GOURI:

• **Natural Rejuvenation**: By stimulating the body's own collagen production, GOURI provides a natural-looking enhancement without adding excessive volume.

• **Minimal Downtime**: Most patients experience mild swelling or redness post-procedure, which typically resolves within a few days, allowing for a quick return to daily activities.

• **Safety Profile**: As a biocompatible and biodegradable product, GOURI integrates seamlessly with the body's tissues, minimizing the risk of adverse reactions.

GOURI represents a significant advancement in aesthetic medicine, offering a non-surgical option for individuals seeking to rejuvenate their skin by harnessing the body's natural regenerative processes. Consultation with a qualified aesthetic practitioner is essential to determine suitability and develop a personalized treatment plan.

Ellansé

Ellansé is a unique dermal filler that not only provides immediate volume correction but also stimulates the body's natural collagen production, leading to longer-lasting and natural-looking results.

Key Features of Ellansé:

• **Immediate Volume Restoration**: Upon injection, Ellansé provides instant correction of wrinkles and folds, restoring facial volume and contours.

• **Collagen Stimulation**: Beyond immediate effects, Ellansé stimulates the body's own collagen production, enhancing skin elasticity, firmness, and overall quality over time.

• **Long-Lasting Results**: Depending on the specific Ellansé product used, results can last from 18 months up to 3 years, reducing the need for frequent touch-ups.

• **Biocompatible and Biodegradable**: Composed of polycaprolactone (PCL) microspheres suspended in a carboxymethylcellulose (CMC) gel, Ellansé is both biocompatible and biodegradable, ensuring safety and natural integration into the skin.

Treatment Areas:

Ellansé is versatile and can be used to address various facial areas, including:

• Nasolabial folds

• Marionette lines

• Cheek volume loss

- Jawline contouring

- Chin augmentation

- Temple hollows

- Hand rejuvenation

Procedure and Recovery:

The treatment involves injecting Ellansé into the desired areas using fine needles or cannulas. The procedure typically takes about 30 to 45 minutes, depending on the number of areas treated. Most patients experience minimal downtime, with possible mild swelling or redness that usually subsides within a few days.

Safety and Considerations:

Ellansé has a strong safety profile; however, as with any injectable treatment, there are potential side effects, including:

- Redness

- Swelling

- Bruising

- Tenderness at the injection site

These side effects are typically mild and resolve spontaneously within a few days. Rare but serious complications, such as vascular occlusion, have been reported; thus, it is crucial to have the procedure performed by a qualified and experienced medical professional.

Why Choose One Over the Other?

For Full-Face Rejuvenation & Gradual Volume: → Sculptra (Best for global collagen stimulation)

For Instant Lift with Long-Term Collagen Boost: → Radiesse (Gives immediate structure & tightens skin)

For Skin Tightening & Subtle Refinement: → Gouri (Best for mild laxity & fine lines without adding bulk)

For Long-Lasting Structural Support & Contouring: → Ellansé (Acts as a filler with collagen-stimulating benefits)

Juvelook and Lenisna are advanced injectable treatments designed to rejuvenate the skin by stimulating collagen production. Both products combine Poly-D,L-lactic acid (PDLLA) with non-cross-linked hyaluronic acid (HA), offering both immediate hydration and long-term skin improvement.

Juvelook:

- **Composition**: Contains 42.5 mg of PDLLA and 7.5 mg of HA, with particle sizes ranging from 10 to 40 micrometers.

- **Application**: Suitable for addressing fine lines, improving skin texture, treating under-eye concerns, and reducing acne scars.

- **Injection Depth**: Administered into the dermis to superficial subcutaneous layers.

- **Results**: Typically visible around two weeks after treatment and can last between 12 to 16 months.

Lenisna:

- **Composition**: Contains 170 mg of PDLLA and 30 mg of HA, with particle sizes between 50 to 60 micrometers.

- **Application**: Effective for treating deep wrinkles, volume loss in the face or hands, and significant tissue defects.

- **Injection Depth**: Targeted at the superficial subcutaneous layer.

- **Results**: Effects appear after about two weeks and can last approximately 18 to 24 months.

Both treatments work by gradually absorbing into the skin, activating fibroblasts to stimulate the production of collagen and elastin, leading to improved skin elasticity and firmness. The choice between Juvelook and Lenisna depends on individual skin concerns and desired outcomes.

Ariessence™ Pure PDGF+: A Next-Gen Biostimulant

Among the evolving range of biostimulants making waves in aesthetic medicine, Ariessence™ Pure PDGF+ stands out as a groundbreaking innovation. Rooted in advanced regenerative science, this treatment harnesses the power of Platelet-Derived Growth Factor (PDGF)—a potent signaling protein that plays a pivotal role in tissue regeneration, collagen synthesis, and cellular communication.

Unlike traditional autologous treatments such as Platelet-Rich Plasma (PRP), which depend on the variability of the patient's own platelets, Ariessence delivers pharmaceutical-grade, recombinant PDGF in a highly purified and consistent format. This ensures predictability, potency, and safety—key components in achieving reliable clinical outcomes.

What Makes Ariessence Unique?

- **Ultra-Purified Formula**: With only four ingredients, Ariessence's formulation eliminates unnecessary additives and focuses on delivering bioactive growth factors at an unparalleled level of purity.

- **Potency**: According to the manufacturer, Ariessence boasts up to 300,000 times the concentration of growth factors found in typical PRP preparations—an extraordinary leap in therapeutic strength.

- **Consistency**: Because it is lab-engineered rather than patient-derived, it removes variability between individuals, offering more uniform outcomes across diverse skin types and conditions.

- **Clinical Heritage**: PDGF has been extensively studied and utilized in medical-grade wound healing and tissue repair, with a strong safety profile and FDA approval in other therapeutic categories.

Treatment Applications

Ariessence can be used as a standalone injectable treatment or combined with microneedling, RF microneedling, laser resurfacing, or dermal fillers. Its regenerative capabilities make it ideal for addressing:

- Skin laxity

- Fine lines and wrinkles

- Dull or uneven skin tone

- Post-procedural recovery

- Acne scarring

Who Is It For?

Ariessence is particularly well-suited to clients seeking visible skin rejuvenation without volumizing, such as those wary of hyaluronic acid fillers but still desiring a refreshed, youthful appearance. It's also excellent for younger patients focused on prevention and mature clients looking for firming and texture improvement.

Comparative Chart Ariessence with Natural Biostimulant PRP, Synthetic Bio stimulant Sculptra.

Feature	Ariessence Pure PDGF+	PRP (Platelet-Rich Plasma)	Sculptra (Poly-L-lactic Acid)
Source	Lab-engineered PDGF (non-autologous)	Autologous (patient's own blood)	Synthetic poly-L-lactic acid (biodegradable polymer)
Key Action	Regenerative signaling for collagen and cell renewal	Moderate collagen stimulation and healing via growth factors	Strong fibroblast stimulation via inflammatory cascade
Onset of Results	Visible results within 2 to 4 weeks	4 to 6 weeks	Gradual, 8 to 12 weeks
Duration	Several months (varies depending on treatment plan)	Typically 3to 6 months	Up to 2 years or longer with full course
Consistency	Highly consistent lab-purified and controlled	Variables depends on patients platelet concentration	Consistent once injected correctly
Texture & Volume	No volume; improves tone, firmness, clarity	Little to no volume; more regenerative	Volumizing effect as collagen builds
Ideal For	Skin quality, texture, early aging, post-laser or microneedling	Prevention, healing, dullness, hair loss	Volume loss, deep folds, structural rejuvenation
Contraindications	Very fewer non-autologous, no allergy risk	Autoimmune disorders, anemia, low platelet counts	History of keloids, active inflammation
Treatment Comfort	Mild topical or needle-based application	Blood draw + microinjections or microneedling	Deep dermal injections; requires massage post-treatment

Product	Main Ingredient	Mechanism of Action	Best For	Longevity
Sculptra	Poly-L-Lactic Acid (PLLA)	Stimulates deep collagen production for gradual volume restoration	Global volume loss, hollow cheeks, temples, buttocks augmentation	Up to 2 yrs
Radiesse	Calcium Hydroxylapatite (CaHA)	Provides immediate lift & stimulates collagen production	Jawline contouring, cheek augmentation, hand rejuvenation	12-18 m
Gouri	Liquid polycaprolactone (PCL)	Fully liquid form spreads evenly to stimulate collagen	Skin laxity, fine lines, overall skill tightening	6-12 m
Ellansé	Polycaprolactone (PCL) microspheres in CMC gel	Immediate volume correction + collagen stimulation for long term skin support	Facial contouring, deep folds, chin & Jawline enhancement	1 to 4 yrs
Profhilo Structura	Hybrid Cooperative Complex (HCC) HA	Hydrates deeply while stimulating collagen, elastin & adipose tissue for skin tighten and volume restoration	Skin laxity, fine lines, overall skin firmness & elasticity	6-12 m
Juvelook	Poly-D,L-lactic acid (PDLLA) and non-cross-linked Hyaluronic Acid (HA)	HA provides immediate hydration and plumping; PDLLA stimulates collagen production for long-term skin rejuvenation	Fine lines, wrinkles, acne scars, skin hydration, peri-orbital rejuvenation	24 m
Lenisna	Poly-D,L-lactic acid (PDLLA) and Hyaluronic Acid (HA)	HA offers immediate volume; PDLLA acts as a collagen stimulator, enhancing skin elasticity and firmness over time	Deep wrinkles, facial volume loss, skin laxity, body rejuvenation	2 yrs
Ariessence	Poly D,L-lactic acid (PDLLA) + Hyaluronic Acid (HA)	PDLLA stimulates type I&III Collagen via a controlled inf. response, HA Provides hydration and elasticity	Under eyes, cheeks, temples, jawline	12-18 m

Biostimulants Guide

What Is Collagen?

Collagen is the most abundant structural protein in the human body. It provides firmness, strength, and elasticity to the skin, and is also a major component of bones, tendons, ligaments, and connective tissue. From our mid-20s, natural collagen production begins to decline—accelerated by sun exposure, smoking, poor diet, and stress—leading to visible signs of ageing such as skin laxity, fine lines, and volume loss.

Cosmetic biostimulant treatments aim to reawaken the body's natural collagen production, resulting in gradual, long-lasting rejuvenation.

Types of Collagen Relevant to Aesthetics

While there are 28 different types of collagen in the body, only a few are relevant when it comes to skin health and aesthetics:

Type I Collagen: The most abundant type, found in skin, tendons, bones, and ligaments. It provides tensile strength and structure.

Type III Collagen: Often found alongside Type I. It plays a key role in the early stages of wound healing and is abundant in youthful skin.

Type IV Collagen: Found in the skin's basement membrane, supporting cell layers and filtration.

Most collagen-inducing injectables used in aesthetics target the stimulation of Type I and Type III collagen.

What Types of Collagen Do Biostimulants Stimulate?

Different biostimulants stimulate collagen at varying depths and rates. Below is a summary of popular collagen-stimulating injectables:

Sculptra (Poly-L-lactic acid): Stimulates Type I collagen. Results begin to appear after 6 to 12 weeks, with full effects developing over several months. Typically requires a series of 2 to 3 treatments, spaced 4 to 6 weeks apart. Longevity: up to 2 to 3 years.

Radiesse (Calcium Hydroxylapatite): Stimulates Type I & III collagen. Offers immediate volume from its carrier gel, with collagen forming over 8 to 12 weeks. Longevity: 12 to 18 months.

Lenisna (Hybrid PLLA + HA): Stimulates Type I and III collagen. Begins working within 6 to 8 weeks and continues to improve skin quality over time. Longevity: 12 to 24 months.

Gouri (Liquid PLLA): A fully solubilised PLLA that spreads evenly. Stimulates Type I and III collagen. Onset around 4 to 6 weeks. Longevity: 6 to 12 months.

Ariessence (Polycaprolactone or PCL): A newer biostimulant that also targets Type I and III collagen. Results typically start after 8 to 10 weeks. Longevity: up to 24 months or more.

How Long Does It Take for Collagen to Form?

Collagen production typically begins around 4 to 8 weeks post-treatment, with visible improvements continuing to build up over 3 to 6 months. This delayed onset is why biostimulants require patience but reward consistency.

Hyperdilution: What Is It and Why Use It?

Hyperdilution involves mixing a biostimulant product with saline and/or lidocaine to reduce its thickness and allow for even spread across a larger treatment area. This technique is ideal when the goal is skin tightening or improving texture, rather than volume restoration.

Products that can be hyperdiluted include:

Radiesse: Commonly hyperdiluted for treating neck, décolletage, arms, buttocks, and thighs to improve skin firmness and crepey texture.

Sculptra: Can be diluted for broader collagen stimulation, such as buttocks or large surface areas like the chest.

Lenisna: May be diluted for superficial collagen induction and skin quality improvement.

Ariessence: Although newer, clinicians are adapting it for dilution-based use in larger treatment zones.

How Do You Choose the Right Biostimulant?

Choosing the appropriate product depends on several factors: skin condition, area treated, desired result, patient tolerance for downtime, and treatment goals.

Here's a simplified guide:

For volume and deep collagen induction: Sculptra or undiluted Radiesse , Ellanse.

For skin tightening and texture improvement: Hyperdiluted Radiesse, Ariessence, and Sculptra.

For subtle, natural glow and hydration: Gouri or Lenisna

For long-lasting collagen stimulation: Ariessence or Sculptra

It's essential to match the product not only to the indication but also to the injector's experience and the patient's expectations.

PRX-T33 Non-Invasive Biostimulant:

PRX-T33 is a next-generation, non-invasive skin biostimulator designed to rejuvenate and revitalize the skin without causing peeling or significant downtime. Unlike traditional chemical peels that focus on exfoliation and resurfacing, PRX-T33 works at a deeper level to stimulate the skin's natural regenerative processes. It is applied topically in a clinical setting and is often referred to as a "peel without peeling" due to its ability to deliver results without visible flaking or irritation.

What Does PRX-T33 Stimulate?

This treatment stimulates fibroblast activity, which plays a key role in collagen production, skin hydration, and overall tissue repair. The active ingredients penetrate the dermis without disrupting the outer skin barrier, prompting cellular renewal, dermal remodelling, and enhanced hydration. The result is improved skin texture, elasticity, and firmness.

Key benefits include:

• Increased collagen and elastin production for firmer skin

• Enhanced hydration without causing dryness

• Reduction in fine lines, wrinkles, and superficial scarring

• Improvement in pigmentation and skin tone

• Tighter pores and a more radiant complexion

How Is It Different from Skin Peels?

Unlike conventional skin peels that work by exfoliating the epidermis (outer skin layer), PRX-T33 is a biostimulatory treatment that bypasses the epidermis and works within the dermis. It does not cause significant peeling or downtime while still achieving deep rejuvenation.

• **No visible peeling**: Traditional chemical peels cause layers of skin to shed, leading to downtime. PRX-T33 stimulates skin renewal without excessive flaking or irritation.

• **Non-ablative**: It does not damage the epidermis, unlike aggressive peels that require recovery time.

• **Stronger regenerative action**: The formulation activates fibroblast cells, leading to long-term skin improvements beyond surface exfoliation.

• **Can be used year-round**: Many chemical peels require caution in summer due to photosensitivity risks, whereas PRX-T33 is safe even in warmer months.

Mode of Action: How Does PRX-T33 Work?
PRX-T33 is a patented formula that combines trichloroacetic acid (TCA) at 33%, hydrogen peroxide (H_2O_2), and kojic acid. Each component plays a specific role:

1. Trichloroacetic Acid (TCA, 33%)

• Traditionally used in peels, but in this formulation, it penetrates the dermis without damaging the epidermis.

• Stimulates fibroblasts to increase collagen production and skin renewal.

• Helps with wrinkles, sagging, and scars.

2. Hydrogen Peroxide (H_2O_2)

• Modulates the action of TCA, preventing excessive peeling.

• Promotes growth factor release and speeds up skin regeneration.

• Has an antiseptic and anti-inflammatory effect.

3. Kojic Acid

• Helps to brighten and even out skin tone, reducing hyperpigmentation.

• Works as a melanin inhibitor, making it beneficial for treating sun spots and post-inflammatory pigmentation.

The treatment is massaged into the skin by a professional using a specific technique to ensure deep penetration. The skin absorbs the product quickly, activating collagen synthesis and tissue remodelling from within.

What to Expect:

PRX-T33 delivers instant and progressive results, meaning the skin looks fresher and more hydrated after just one session, but the full benefits build up over multiple treatments.

Immediate effects (after 1 session):

firmer, plumper skin

A visible glow and improved hydration

Tighter pores

Long-term effects (after a full course):

Increased collagen and elastin production

Reduction in fine lines, wrinkles, and mild sagging

Improved skin tone and texture

Reduction in pigmentation, sun spots, and acne scars

Since the treatment does not cause flaking or downtime, clients can return to their normal activities immediately after.

How Many Treatments Are Needed?

For optimal results, a course of 4–6 sessions is typically recommended, spaced one week apart. The exact number of sessions depends on the skin concern being treated.

• For general skin rejuvenation → 4 sessions

• For deeper wrinkles, scars, or hyperpigmentation → 5–6 sessions

• For acne-prone or dull skin → 3–4 sessions

Many clients opt for maintenance treatments every few months to prolong the effects. PRX-T33 is often combined with other treatments like microneedling, RF skin tightening, or PRP to enhance its benefits.

Is PRX-T33 FM (For Men)?

Yes! PRX-T33 is suitable for both men and women who want to improve their skin without undergoing aggressive treatments. Since it doesn't involve needles or visible peeling, it's an excellent choice for men who prefer a non-invasive, low-maintenance approach to skin rejuvenation.

PRX-T33 is a powerful yet gentle alternative to traditional peels, offering deep skin rejuvenation with no peeling, no pain, and no downtime. By stimulating collagen and fibroblast activity without damaging the surface layer, it provides an effective, year-round skin solution for those looking to enhance their complexion naturally.

CHAPTER 34: USING YOUR OWN CELLS TO REJUVENATE

PRP, PRF, and PRP Filler (Cellenis)

Regenerative medicine has brought ground breaking advancements in aesthetics, with platelet-derived treatments like PRP (Platelet-Rich Plasma), PRF (Platelet-Rich Fibrin), and PRP Filler (Plasma Biofiller) offering natural ways to restore volume, improve skin quality, and stimulate tissue repair. These treatments use your own blood to harness the power of platelets and growth factors, making them a powerful tool in aesthetic and anti-aging treatments.

What Are They?

1. PRP (Platelet-Rich Plasma)

PRP is a concentrated plasma solution derived from your blood, rich in growth factors and platelets. It has been widely used in aesthetic medicine, orthopedics, and wound healing to stimulate collagen production, tissue repair, and overall skin rejuvenation.

2. PRF (Platelet-Rich Fibrin)

PRF is a more advanced version of PRP, containing a fibrin matrix that allows for a slower release of growth factors. This means longer-lasting stimulation of healing and collagen production. Unlike PRP, PRF is obtained without anticoagulants, which results in a thicker, gel-like consistency.

3. PRP Filler (Plasma Biofiller) - Cellenis

PRP Filler, also called Plasma Biofiller, is a thickened version of PRP achieved by heating plasma to create a gel-like consistency. This allows it to act as a natural filler, providing temporary volume while also delivering regenerative benefits.

What is the Difference?

Features	PRP	PRF	PRP Filler
Growth Factor Release	Immediate	Sustained (slow release)	Slow release + volume effect
Consistency	Liquid	Gel-like	Thickened gel (filler-like)
Longevity	Short-term (1-2 weeks)	Longer-lasting (2-4 weeks)	Temporary volume (3-6 months)
Anticoagulants	Yes (prevents clotting)	No (allows natural clotting)	No (plasma thickened by heat)

Use Skin rejuvenation, hair restoration Wound healing, collagen production Facial volume, contouring, regenerative benefits

Purpose of All Three Treatments

PRP: Improves skin texture, boosts collagen, accelerates healing, and is commonly used for hair restoration and facial rejuvenation.

PRF: Provides a longer-lasting release of growth factors, making it ideal for skin rejuvenation, under-eye hollows, and wound healing.

PRP Filler (Plasma Biofiller): Acts as a natural dermal filler while delivering regenerative properties, making it suitable for volume loss in areas like cheeks, nasolabial folds, and lips.

How Do You Get PRP?

1. A small amount of blood is drawn from your arm.

2. The blood is spun in a centrifuge to separate the platelets and plasma from red and white blood cells.

3. The platelet-rich plasma is extracted and used for treatment.

How Do You Get PRF?

1. Blood is drawn from the patient.

2. The blood is centrifuged at a lower speed and for a shorter time than PRP to preserve fibrin and white blood cells.

3. Since no anticoagulant is used, the PRF forms a clot-like gel that is then applied to the treatment area.

How Do You Get PRP Filler?

1. PRP is obtained using the same process as standard PRP.

2. The plasma is then heated at a controlled temperature, causing it to thicken into a gel-like consistency.

3. Once cooled, it is ready for injection as a natural volumizer.

What Do They Do in the Body?

PRP: Stimulates collagen production, enhances tissue repair, and promotes healing.

PRF: Releases growth factors slowly over time, leading to prolonged regenerative effects.

PRP Filler: Provides immediate volume and stimulates collagen while gradually being absorbed by the body.

Which One to Choose & Why?

Choose PRP if you want a quick boost in collagen production, skin rejuvenation, or hair restoration without volume enhancement.

Choose PRF if you want a longer-lasting effect with sustained growth factor release, particularly for delicate areas like the under-eyes.

Choose PRP Filler (Plasma Biofiller) if you need both volume replacement and regenerative benefits, making it ideal for areas of volume loss.

Each treatment has its strengths, and the best choice depends on your goals whether it is rejuvenation, repair, or natural volume restoration. By using your own cells, these treatments provide a safe, effective, and natural approach to maintaining youthful, healthy skin.

Treatment	What is it	Indications of Use	How Long Does it Last	How Many Treatments
PRP (Platelet-Rich Plasma)	A concentration of platelets from your own blood, spun at high speed to separate plasma rich in growth factors.	Skin rejuvenation, fine lines, texture, acne scars, hair restoration.	3–6 months (biological stimulation, not volumizing).	Initial series of 3–4 treatments spaced 4–6 weeks apart, then maintenance 1–2 times/year.
PRF (Platelet-Rich Fibrin)	Second-generation PRP, spun at lower speeds, no anticoagulant, forming a fibrin matrix that slowly releases growth factors.	Under-eye hollows, fine lines, crepey skin, early volume loss, slow-healing areas.	Up to 12 months (longer release of growth factors).	2–4 sessions spaced 6–8 weeks apart, then 1–2 annually.
PRP Filler (Bio-filler / Plasma Gel)	Heated PRP converted into a gel consistency and injected like a filler for volume.	Tear troughs, cheeks, nasolabial folds, lips, skin creping, facial hollows.	3–6 months (depends on technique and patient).	1–2 sessions initially; may repeat every 3–6 months for volume

CHAPTER 35: BIO-FILLER

In the evolving landscape of aesthetic medicine, the quest for natural and effective rejuvenation techniques has led to the development of autologous treatments those utilizing the patient's own biological materials. One such innovation is the Platelet-Rich Plasma (PRP) Bio-Filler, a treatment that serves both as a dermal filler and a biostimulant, offering a holistic approach to facial rejuvenation.

Understanding PRP Bio-Filler

PRP Bio-Filler is an advanced aesthetic procedure that harnesses the regenerative properties of a patient's blood to restore facial volume and enhance skin quality. Unlike traditional synthetic fillers, this method reduces the risk of allergic reactions and ensures better biocompatibility.

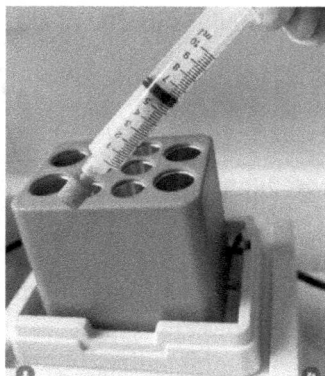

Platelet poor plasma is heated and the albumin thickens. Once it cools Platelet Rich Plasma is mixed with the Platelet Poor plasma and forms a bio stimulating filler.

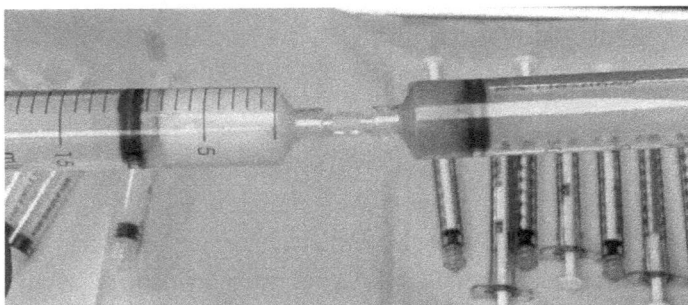

Thickened PPP mixed with PRP to make biofiller.

Application and Benefits

PRP Bio-Filler is versatile and can be used in various facial regions, with notable efficacy in treating tear trough deformities:

Tear Trough Rejuvenation: The under-eye area often exhibits signs of aging, such as hollowness and dark circles. Injecting PRP Bio-Filler into this region not only restores volume but also stimulates collagen production, leading to improved skin texture and elasticity. This dual action addresses both the superficial and underlying causes of under-eye concerns.

Duration and Longevity

The effects of PRP Bio-Filler are both immediate and progressive:

Immediate Results: Post-injection, patients may notice an instant improvement in volume and skin tightness.

Long-Term Benefits: The biostimulatory properties of the filler promote ongoing collagen synthesis and tissue regeneration.

Typically, the results can last between 3 to 6 months, with some variations based on individual factors such as age, skin condition, and lifestyle.

Advantages over Traditional Fillers

PRP Bio-Filler offers several benefits compared to conventional dermal fillers:

Natural Composition: Utilizing the patient's own blood eliminates the risk of allergic reactions and ensures high biocompatibility.

Dual Functionality: It acts as a filler to restore volume and as a biostimulant to enhance skin quality intrinsically.

Safety Profile: The autologous nature of the treatment minimizes potential complications associated with synthetic fillers.

PRF vs Cellenis® Derma Filler: Natural Healing vs Structural Support

Platelet-Rich Fibrin (PRF) and Cellenis® DermaFiller both harness the regenerative power of the patient's own blood, but they serve different purposes in aesthetic medicine.

- **PRF** forms a natural fibrin clot after injection. This clot acts as a short-lived scaffold that supports wound healing, collagen production, and tissue repair. It is fully metabolised within 5–10 days, making it ideal for stimulating the skin's natural rejuvenation processes without adding volume.

- **Cellenis® DermaFiller** on the other hand, forms a proteinic scaffold—a more durable structure designed to mimic the body's extracellular matrix. This scaffold supports cell regeneration while also providing immediate volume and structural lift, especially useful in delicate areas like the tear troughs. It remains active in the tissue for 3 to 6 months, offering both regenerative and volumising effects.

In summary:

- **PRF** = Temporary fibrin matrix for healing and collagen boost

- **Cellenis DermaFiller** = Longer-lasting protein scaffold for regeneration + volume

PRF vs Cellenis® DermaFiller Comparison

Feature	PRF (Platelet-Rich Fibrin)	Cellenis® DermaFiller
Type of Structure	Fibrin Clot	Proteinic Scaffold
Primary Function	Stimulate healing & collagen production	Regeneration + structural support
Composition	Natural fibrin from blood	Engineered protein matrix
Duration in Tissue	5-10 days	3-6 Months
Mechanism of Action	Forms clot post-injection; supports natural repair	Scaffold integrates with tissue, supports regeneration
Best Used For	Skin texture, fine lines, crepey skin	Tear troughs, volume restoration, support
Volume Effect	No immediate volume	Immediate volume + lift

Why Cellenis® DermaFiller

- Induce new collagen to form and enhance skin radiance and revitalization
- Effective for face and body rejuvenation
- Derived from completely autologous materials
- Decelerate aging by immediately replacing missing volume while bio-stimulating to prevent further tissue lost
- One kit provides 13ml of regenerative material for a comprehensive treatment.

How Cellenis Dermal Filler is Created – In Simple Terms

Cellenis Dermal Filler is made from your own blood, so it's completely natural and unique to you. Here's how it works:

1.   A small blood sample is taken – just like having a routine blood test.

2.   The blood goes into a special tube designed to separate its components.

3.   We spin the tube in a centrifuge – this rapid spinning separates the blood into layers:

•   Platelet Poor Plasma (PPP) – the clearer top layer, which we can transform into a gel.

•   Platelet Rich Plasma (PRP) – the golden layer rich in growth factors and healing platelets.

4.   The PPP is gently heated – this changes its texture from a liquid into a smooth, gel-like consistency (about 8 mls).

5.   The PRP is collected – usually around 3 mls of this powerful, rejuvenating liquid.

6.   The two are combined – the PRP is mixed back into the PPP gel. This creates a natural filler that is rich in your own platelets.

The end result is a bio-filler that not only restores volume but also stimulates your skin's natural rejuvenation process — improving texture, tone, and overall vitality over time.

Because it's made from your own blood, the risk of allergic reaction is extremely low, and you're giving your skin a boost from the inside out.

Conclusion

PRP Bio-Filler represents a significant advancement in aesthetic treatments, merging the benefits of dermal fillers with the regenerative potential of biostimulants. Its natural composition, combined with its efficacy in areas like the tear troughs, makes it a compelling option for individuals seeking holistic facial rejuvenation. As with any medical procedure, it is essential to consult with qualified healthcare professionals to determine suitability and ensure optimal outcomes.

CHAPTER 36: SKIN BOOSTERS

Skin boosters are a revolutionary class of injectable treatments designed to enhance skin hydration, elasticity, and overall appearance without adding significant volume. By delivering vital substances directly into the skin, these treatments address various concerns, from fine lines to uneven texture.

What Are Skin Boosters?

Skin boosters are minimally invasive procedures that involve injecting hydrating and nourishing substances, such as hyaluronic acid (HA), amino acids, vitamins, and polynucleotides, into the dermal layer of the skin. Unlike traditional dermal fillers that add volume, skin boosters focus on improving skin quality by:

Enhancing Hydration: Attracting and retaining moisture within the skin.

Stimulating Collagen Production: Encouraging the natural synthesis of collagen and elastin.

Improving Elasticity and Firmness: Restoring a youthful bounce to the skin.

Smoothing Fine Lines and Wrinkles: Reducing the appearance of superficial aging signs.

Popular Skin Booster Treatments

Here are some notable skin booster treatments, their compositions, injection techniques, and expected results:

1. Profhilo

Composition: Profhilo contains one of the highest concentrations of pure hyaluronic acid (64 mg/2 ml) without any chemical cross-linking agents.

Injection Technique: Administered using the Bio-Aesthetic Points (BAP) technique, which involves injecting small amounts into specific points on the face to ensure even distribution and optimal results.

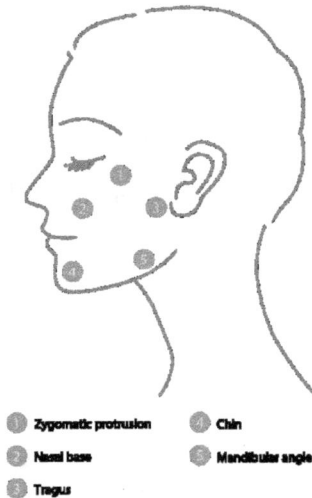

1. Zygomatic protrusion   4. Chin
2. Nasal base   5. Mandibular angle
3. Tragus

Results: Patients often notice improved skin hydration, elasticity, and a subtle lifting effect within a few weeks. A typical protocol involves two sessions spaced four weeks apart.

2. Jalupro

Composition: A blend of hyaluronic acid and amino acids, including glycine, l-proline, l-lysine, and l-leucine, which are essential for collagen synthesis.

Injection Technique: Injected into the superficial to mid-dermal layer using fine needles, targeting areas with signs of aging or dehydration.

Results: Enhances skin texture, reduces fine lines, and promotes a radiant complexion. Multiple sessions may be recommended for optimal outcomes.

3. NCTF 135 HA (Filorga)

Composition: A mesotherapy solution containing hyaluronic acid and a cocktail of 59 other ingredients, including vitamins, minerals, amino acids, and antioxidants.

Injection Technique: Micro-injections are administered superficially across the treatment area to deliver the solution directly into the dermis.

Results: Improved skin hydration, brightness, and elasticity, with a reduction in fine lines and an overall rejuvenated appearance.

4. Rejuran

Composition: Contains polynucleotides (PN) derived from salmon DNA, known for their regenerative properties.

Injection Technique: Administered through micro-injections into the dermis, focusing on areas requiring rejuvenation.

Results: Promotes skin healing, improves elasticity, and reduces fine lines. A series of treatments is often recommended for best results.

5. Skinvive

Composition: A hyaluronic acid-based injectable designed specifically for skin quality improvement.

Injection Technique: Injected into the mid to deep dermis using fine needles, covering the entire treatment area.

Results: Provides deep hydration, enhances elasticity, and smooths fine lines, with effects lasting up to nine months.

6. Restylane Skinboosters

Composition: Stabilized hyaluronic acid formulated to improve skin quality.

Injection Technique: Micro-injections are evenly distributed across the treatment area, delivering HA into the dermis.

Results: Enhances skin hydration, elasticity, and smoothness, leading to a refreshed and radiant appearance.

Injection Techniques

The success of skin booster treatments largely depends on the injection technique, which ensures even distribution and minimizes discomfort. Common methods include:

Micro-Injections: Using fine needles to administer small amounts of the product across the treatment area.

Cannula Technique: Utilizing a blunt-tipped cannula to deliver the product with minimal entry points, reducing the risk of bruising.

Bio-Aesthetic Points (BAP): A specialized technique used in treatments like Profhilo, targeting specific points to maximize efficacy and distribution.

A topical anaesthetic is often applied before the procedure to enhance patient comfort.

8. Sunekos

Regenerative Skin Support Without Volume

Sunekos is often grouped under the term "skin booster," but that description is incomplete.

It is not simply a hydrating injectable.

Sunekos is a regenerative treatment designed to support fibroblast function and improve the extracellular matrix — without adding volume.

That distinction is critical.

It does not inflate tissue.

It strengthens it.

What Makes Sunekos Different?

Traditional skin boosters typically contain hyaluronic acid alone. Their primary effect is hydration and temporary plumping.

Sunekos combines:

Hyaluronic acid

A patented amino acid complex

The amino acids include:

Glycine

L-Proline

L-Lysine

L-Alanine

L-Valine

These are essential building blocks for collagen and elastin synthesis.

This specific formulation is designed to stimulate fibroblast activity — the cells responsible for producing:

Collagen

Elastin

Fibronectin

Rather than filling the face, Sunekos improves dermal biology.

It supports regeneration.

It does not create projection.

Understanding Fibroblasts and Cellular Senescence

Fibroblasts are the structural cells within the dermis.

With age, fibroblasts:

Slow down

Produce less collagen

Become less responsive

Enter a state known as cellular senescence

Cellular senescence refers to aged cells that no longer function efficiently and contribute to tissue degeneration.

Sunekos helps support fibroblast function by providing the biochemical environment needed for collagen production and dermal repair.

It supports the structure of the skin — without volumising it.

Sunekos Performa

Sunekos Performa contains:

Low molecular weight hyaluronic acid

The amino acid complex described above

It is designed for delicate areas and early ageing.

Ideal areas:

Under-eye region

Upper eyelids (carefully selected cases)

Neck

Décolletage

Fine lines

Performa improves:

Skin thickness

Elasticity

Crepiness

Fine lines

It does not fill hollows.

It improves the quality of the skin covering them.

Sunekos 1200

Sunekos 1200 contains:

Higher molecular weight hyaluronic acid

The same amino acid complex

The higher molecular weight component provides greater dermal support and tissue reinforcement.

It is better suited to areas with more advanced dermal depletion.

Common areas:

Midface skin quality

Lower face

Jawline region

Areas of collagen loss

Sunekos 1200 does not act as filler.

It does not lift or sculpt.

It strengthens and supports dermal integrity.

Can Sunekos Be Used Under the Eyes?

Yes — and this is one of its most valuable applications.

Under-eye ageing is often due to:

Skin thinning

Reduced elasticity

Early collagen decline

Mild hollowing

Using filler alone in thin under-eye skin can create heaviness.

Sunekos Performa improves:

Dermal thickness

Fine crepiness

Elasticity

Brightness

It enhances tissue quality without adding weight.

How Is Sunekos Injected?

Sunekos is typically administered using:

Small micro-deposits

Linear threading techniques

Strategic dermal placement

It is injected into the dermis to stimulate fibroblast activity.

It is not placed as a bolus for projection.

A typical course includes:

Three to four sessions

Two weeks apart

Results develop gradually as collagen production improves.

What Sunekos Does and Does Not Do

Sunekos can:

Improve skin elasticity

Enhance hydration

Support collagen production

Improve dermal thickness

Reduce fine lines

Support fibroblast function

Sunekos does not:

Add facial projection

Replace dermal filler

Lift cheeks

Reshape contours

Create jawline definition

It is regenerative support, not volumisation.

When Not to Use Sunekos

Understanding its limits is essential.

Sunekos is not appropriate when:

Significant structural volume loss is present

Advanced cheek collapse requires projection

Deep tear trough hollowing needs structural correction

Severe lower face heaviness requires lifting strategies

It is not suitable for patients seeking:

Immediate dramatic results

Facial sculpting

Projection or contour enhancement

Sunekos improves skin quality.

It does not replace filler where structure is missing.

It should not be used in areas of:

Active infection

Active herpes outbreak

Inflamed skin

Known hypersensitivity to ingredients

The Balanced Approach

The most common mistake in aesthetics is treating lines before structure.

The second most common mistake is adding volume without improving skin quality.

Sunekos works best when integrated into a long-term strategy:

Structure when needed

Regeneration always

Maintenance consistently

It represents a shift in modern aesthetics:

From filling

To regenerating

From inflating

To strengthening

From chasing lines

To supporting biology

That is responsible rejuvenation.

9. Tesoro Collagen

Tesoro Collagen is an injectable skin booster designed to improve skin quality by supporting collagen regeneration rather than adding volume. It belongs to the newer generation of regenerative aesthetic treatments that focus on skin health, texture, and resilience.

What Makes Tesoro Collagen Different

Tesoro Collagen is formulated with recombinant human-like collagen (RHLC). This collagen is laboratory-engineered to closely replicate the structure of natural human collagen, unlike older collagen products derived from animal sources. Because it mimics the body's own collagen, it integrates well into the dermis and is associated with a lower risk of allergic reactions or inflammatory responses.

Rather than acting as a traditional filler, Tesoro Collagen works by supporting the extracellular matrix, encouraging fibroblast activity and improving the skin's natural regenerative processes.

How It Works in the Skin

When injected into the dermis, Tesoro Collagen helps to:

- Improve skin firmness and elasticity
- Enhance hydration and skin texture
- Support collagen synthesis over time
- Improve skin quality rather than alter facial shape

Results develop gradually, as the skin responds biologically to stimulation, making this treatment ideal for patients seeking natural, subtle rejuvenation.

Areas Commonly Treated

Tesoro Collagen is particularly well suited to delicate and thin-skinned areas, including:

- Under-eye region
- Face (fine lines and crepey skin)

- Neck and décolletage

- Hands

It may also be used to improve overall skin quality in patients with early signs of ageing or loss of dermal density.

Treatment Protocol

A typical treatment course involves:

- A series of three sessions, spaced approximately four weeks apart

- Gradual improvement seen after the second session

- Maintenance treatments every six to twelve months, depending on skin condition and ageing factors

Because this is a regenerative treatment, results are progressive rather than immediate.

Key Ingredients and Skin Benefits

In addition to recombinant human-like collagen, Tesoro Collagen formulations often include:

- Sodium hyaluronate for hydration

- Amino acids essential for collagen synthesis

- Peptides that support skin repair and renewal

- Supporting ingredients that enhance skin tone and vitality

This combination targets both hydration and structural support within the dermis.

Who Is It Best Suited For

Tesoro Collagen is suitable for patients who:

- Want skin rejuvenation without added volume

- Prefer gradual, natural-looking results

- Have early to moderate signs of skin ageing

- Are concerned about skin thinning, fine lines, or loss of elasticity

It is not a replacement for dermal fillers, but rather a complementary treatment within a comprehensive skin rejuvenation plan.

Clinical Considerations

Tesoro Collagen should only be administered by trained medical professionals. As with all injectable treatments, patient selection, correct injection depth, and appropriate technique are essential to achieve optimal outcomes and minimise risk.

Expected Results

Patients can anticipate the following outcomes from skin booster treatments:

Immediate Hydration: Skin appears more hydrated and plump shortly after treatment.

Improved Texture and Elasticity: Over subsequent weeks, the skin becomes smoother and more elastic.

Reduction in Fine Lines: Fine lines and superficial wrinkles diminish, leading to a more youthful appearance.

Enhanced Radiance: Overall skin tone appears more even and luminous.

Results vary based on the specific product used, individual skin conditions, and adherence to the recommended treatment protocol.

In summary, skin boosters offer a versatile and effective solution for individuals seeking to enhance their skin's hydration, texture, and overall vitality.

Skin Booster Comparison Chart

Feature	Tesoro Collagen	Profhilo	NCTF 135	Sunekos
Primary action	Dermal collagen support and regeneration	Hydration-driven bioremodelling	Cellular revitalisation	Collagen and elastin stimulation
Key components	Recombinant human-like collagen	Stabilised hyaluronic acid	Vitamins, amino acids, antioxidants	Hyaluronic acid with amino acids
Volume effect	None	Minimal	None	Minimal
Ideal indications	Crepey skin, dermal thinning	Dehydration, early laxity	Dull, tired skin	Fine lines, early ageing
Common areas	Face, eyes, neck, hands	Face, neck, décolletage	Face, neck, hands	Face, under-eye, neck
Treatment course	3 sessions, 4 weeks apart	2 sessions, 4 weeks apart	3–5 sessions	3 sessions, 7–10 days apart
Downtime	Minimal	Minimal	Minimal	Minimal

CHAPTER 37: EMERGING TRENDS IN AESTHETIC MEDICINE

The field of aesthetic medicine is rapidly evolving, with continuous advancements in injectables, regenerative treatments, and technology-driven solutions. While Korea remains at the forefront of skin innovation, Australia and the USA have strict regulatory frameworks, meaning that many of these cutting-edge treatments are not yet widely available. However, Europe and Korea are leading the way in pioneering new therapies that will likely shape the future of aesthetic medicine.

This chapter explores some of the latest developments, including exosomes, stem cell therapies, AI-driven treatments, non-invasive skin tightening, and the trend toward natural-looking enhancements.

Exosome Therapy : A New Frontier in Skin Rejuvenation

Exosomes are extracellular vesicles that carry proteins, lipids, and genetic material between cells, promoting cell regeneration, repair, and communication. In aesthetic medicine, exosome-based treatments are gaining attention for their potential to improve skin texture, boost collagen, and accelerate wound healing.

Notable Exosome-Based Products & Treatments

Skin Booster Exosome Therapy (Korea) Enhances collagen synthesis, improving elasticity, hydration, and skin tone. Popular in high-end Korean aesthetic clinics.

Platelet Skin Sciences Renewosome Serums (Europe) Uses platelet-derived exosomes to reduce fine lines, wrinkles, and improve hair density.

Rose Stem Cell-Derived Exosomes Under research for their anti-aging effects and ability to promote youthful skin renewal.

Regulatory Considerations: Exosome therapy is still undergoing clinical validation, with varying levels of approval across different countries.

Stem Cell Therapies : The Next Generation of Regenerative Aesthetics. Stem cell treatments harness the body's natural healing abilities for skin rejuvenation, tissue repair, and volume restoration.

Innovations in Stem Cell Aesthetics

Stem Cell Fat Grafting : Uses adipose-derived stem cells (ADSCs) extracted from fat deposits to restore volume in the face, breasts, and hips.

Exosome-Infused Stem Cell Serums Combining exosomes and stem cells to accelerate skin regeneration. While promising, stem cell therapies face regulatory hurdles in many countries due to concerns over safety, consistency, and ethical sourcing.

Artificial Intelligence (AI) in Aesthetics

AI is revolutionizing the diagnosis, treatment planning, and outcome prediction in aesthetic medicine.

AI-Powered Facial Analysis : Software that scans a patients' face to recommend customized treatment plans.

AI-Assisted Injectables Algorithms that help determine the optimal placement of fillers and botulinum toxin for symmetry and balance.

Virtual Try-On Technology : Allows patients to preview their post-treatment results before undergoing procedures.

AI-driven tools will enhance precision and personalize treatments for superior patient outcomes.

Non-Invasive Skin Tightening & Lifting

Patients are increasingly seeking non-surgical alternatives to facelifts, leading to advancements in energy-based treatments:

High-Intensity Focused Ultrasound (HIFU) Stimulates collagen production deep within the skin to provide a lifting effect.

Radiofrequency Microneedling (Morpheus8, Profound RF) Combines microneedling with RF energy to tighten loose skin and improve texture.

Plasma Energy Devices (Jett Plasma, Plexr) Use plasma energy to tighten excess skin, particularly for non-surgical eyelid lifts. These treatments offer minimal downtime while still delivering visible improvements in skin laxity.

Combination Treatments & Treatments Stacking

The trend of stacking multiple treatments in a single session is gaining popularity. Combining injectables, lasers, and regenerative therapies can address multiple concerns at once for more comprehensive results.

Example of Treatment Stacking:

PRP (Platelet-Rich Plasma) + RF Microneedling = Boosts collagen remodelling & skin tightening.

Exosome Therapy + Skin Boosters = Enhances hydration & cellular repair.

Botox + HA Fillers + Bio-Stimulants = Creates a balanced, natural facial rejuvenation.

Why It Works: By combining synergistic treatments, patients achieve better, longer-lasting results with less downtime.

Natural-Looking Enhancements : The Shift Toward Subtlety Modern aesthetic trends emphasize natural beauty over excessive augmentation. Patients are moving away from overfilled, frozen looks and opting for treatments that enhance their unique facial features.

Bio-Stimulants (Sculptra & Radiesse) Stimulate collagen production for gradual, subtle volume restoration.

Microdosing Botox (Baby Botox) Uses smaller amounts of botulinum toxin for a more natural, expressive appearance.

Skin Boosters & Light Fillers Improve skin hydration and elasticity rather than adding bulk.

The future of aesthetics is about refinement, not transformation.

Regenerative Aesthetics : The Future of Beauty & Longevity

The next generation of treatments will move beyond aesthetics to enhancing overall skin health and slowing the aging process at a cellular level.

Exosome Therapy & Stem Cell Infusions Repair and rejuvenate skin from within.

Peptide & Growth Factor Serums Target cell regeneration and skin longevity.

NAD+ & Anti-Aging Supplements Support mitochondrial function and collagen synthesis.

The focus is shifting toward preventative and regenerative solutions rather than simply reversing aging.

Conclusion: The Future of Aesthetic Medicine

Exosomes, stem cell therapies, and AI-driven treatments are shaping the future of aesthetics. Energy-based devices like RF microneedling and HIFU are replacing more invasive procedures. Combination treatments (treatment stacking) enhance results while minimizing downtime. The demand for natural, subtle enhancements is driving innovation in skin boosters, bio-stimulants, and microdosing techniques. Regenerative aesthetics is emerging as the ultimate goal, focusing on long-term skin health and aging prevention.

As research and technology continue to advance, these cutting-edge treatments will become more accessible and refined, paving the way for a new era of aesthetic medicine.

CHAPTER 38: MESODERM INJECTABLE INTERACTIONS & MESOTHERAPY

Mesotherapy is a non-surgical cosmetic procedure that involves injecting a mixture of vitamins, minerals, enzymes, hormones, and plant extracts into the middle layer of the skin, known as the mesoderm. This technique aims to rejuvenate and tighten the skin, as well as remove excess fat.

How different injectables Interact with the Mesodermal Layers of the Skin:

Since the mesoderm gives rise to the dermis and hypodermis, injectables that target these layers aim to stimulate collagen, elastin, and fat production. Here is how various injectables interact with mesoderm-derived skin structures:

1. Hyaluronic Acid (HA) Fillers (e.g., Juvederm, Restylane, Belotero)

Target Layer: Primarily dermis and superficial hypodermis

Mechanism:

HA binds water, hydrating and volumizing the dermis. Cross-linked HA fillers provide structural support but do not directly stimulate mesenchymal stem cells or fibroblasts.

Some newer HA fillers (e.g., **Profhilo, Viscoderm Hydrobooster**) promote collagen synthesis and hydration without excessive volume.

Mesodermal Interaction: Mild stimulation of fibroblasts via mechanical stretching of the extracellular matrix (ECM).

2. Profhilo Structura (Hybrid HA)

Target Layer: Deep dermis & hypodermis (fat compartments)

Mechanism:

HA hybrid complexes create an optimal bio-stimulatory environment. Stimulates adipocyte precursors (mesenchymal stem cells - MSCs), leading to natural fat restoration in atrophic areas. Increases Type I and III collagen and elastin, improving skin quality without adding bulk like traditional fillers.

Mesodermal Interaction: Direct stimulation of MSCs, fibroblasts, and adipocytes for fat regeneration and ECM remodelling.

3. Sculptra (Poly-L-Lactic Acid, PLLA)

Target Layer: Deep dermis & subcutaneous layer

Mechanism:

PLLA microparticles act as a collagen biostimulator, triggering fibroblast activation.

Unlike HA fillers, Sculptra induces neocollagenesis (Type I collagen synthesis) over months. Some studies suggest PLLA may have a minor effect on adipogenesis, but it primarily restores volume by thickening the dermis.

Mesodermal Interaction: Strong fibroblast activation for dermal thickening, but minimal direct impact on adipose tissue.

4. Radiesse (Calcium Hydroxylapatite, CaHA)

Target Layer: Deep dermis & upper hypodermis

Mechanism:

Stimulates fibroblasts to produce collagen and elastin.

The CaHA microspheres act as a scaffold, promoting long-term dermal rejuvenation. Can be diluted for skin-tightening effects or used undiluted for volumization.

Mesodermal Interaction: Significant fibroblast stimulation Neocollagenesis. No direct fat regeneration, but improves structural support.

5. Platelet-Rich Plasma (PRP) & Platelet-Rich Fibrin (PRF)

Target Layer: Dermis & hypodermis

Mechanism:

Growth factors (PDGF, TGF-Î², VEGF) stimulate fibroblasts and adipocyte precursors, leading to collagen synthesis and potential fat restoration. PRP enhances vascularization, improving skin hydration and wound healing.

PRF (a slower-releasing version) may support stem cell differentiation into adipocytes.

Mesodermal Interaction: Direct MSC activation, fibroblast proliferation, and possible adipogenesis stimulation.

6. Exosomes & Stem Cell-Based Injectables (Emerging Therapies)

Target Layer: Dermis & hypodermis

Mechanism:

Exosomes from MSC-derived sources contain growth factors, microRNAs, and proteins that enhance skin regeneration. These therapies have shown promise in stimulating dermal fibroblasts AND inducing adipogenesis, potentially restoring lost fat naturally. Some research suggests that exosomes may promote sustained fat cell differentiation, similar to Profhilo Structura.

Mesodermal Interaction: High potential for fibroblast and fat regeneration but still under clinical evaluation.

Comparison Table: Which Injectables Best Stimulate the Mesoderm

Injectable	Targets Fibroblasts (Collagen Boosting)
HA Fillers (Juvederm, Restylane)	Mild
Profhilo Structura	Moderate-High
Sculptra (PLLA)	Very High
Radiesse (CaHA)	High
PRP/PRF	Moderate- High
Exosomes & Stem Cells	Very High

Final Thoughts: Choosing the Right Treatment Based on Mesodermal Needs

If you want hydration & mild skin tightening , HA-based products **(e.g., Profhilo, Skinboosters)**

If you need volume restoration via collagen stimulation, **Sculptra or Radiesse**

If you want fat regeneration and natural volumization **Profhilo Structura or PRP/Exosomes**

If you need a mix of collagen, elastin, and hydration **Profhilo Structura + Sculptra (stacked treatments)** In mesotherapy, customized "cocktails "are prepared, containing specific active ingredients tailored to address various concerns:

1. Skin Rejuvenation

For enhancing skin quality and appearance, mesotherapy cocktails may include:

Vitamins: Such as vitamin C and E, to promote collagen production and protect against free radicals.

Hyaluronic Acid: To hydrate and plump the skin.

Antioxidants: To combat oxidative stress and improve skin radiance.

These components work synergistically to rejuvenate and tighten the skin.

2. Hair Restoration

Mesotherapy can address hair loss by delivering nutrients directly to the hair follicles. Cocktails for hair restoration may contain:

Vitamins: Such as biotin, to strengthen hair and promote growth.

Amino Acids: To support keratin production.

Minerals: Like zinc and copper, essential for healthy hair follicles.

These injections aim to stimulate blood circulation and provide the necessary nutrients to encourage hair regrowth.

3. Fat Reduction

Mesotherapy is also utilized for body contouring and reducing localized fat deposits. Cocktails designed for fat reduction often include:

Phosphatidylcholine: A phospholipid that aids in breaking down fat cells.

Deoxycholate: A bile salt that emulsifies fat, enhancing its breakdown.

Caffeine: To stimulate metabolism and lipolysis.

These substances work together to break down fat cells, which are then naturally eliminated by the body. Studies have shown that mesotherapy using phosphatidylcholine, alone or combined with organic silicium, can effectively reduce submental fat deposits.

Safety and Considerations

While mesotherapy offers various aesthetic benefits, it's essential to consult with a qualified healthcare professional before undergoing treatment. Potential side effects may include bruising, swelling, and allergic reactions. Ensuring the procedure is performed by an experienced practitioner can minimize risks and enhance outcomes. In summary, mesotherapy is a versatile technique that addresses multiple cosmetic concerns by delivering targeted treatments directly to the mesodermal layer. Whether aiming for skin rejuvenation, hair restoration, or fat reduction, customized mesotherapy cocktails offer a personalized approach to aesthetic enhancement.

CHAPTER 39: THREAD LIFTING, COLLAGEN STIMULATION, AND CONSIDERATIONS FOR LONG-TERM REJUVENATION

Thread lifts have gained popularity as a minimally invasive alternative to facelifts, offering skin tightening and collagen stimulation with minimal downtime. With advancements in technology, thread procedures have evolved from simple skin repositioning to bio-stimulating treatments that improve overall skin quality.

This chapter explores the different types of threads, their longevity, best patient selection, combination treatments, complications, and long-term considerations especially for those considering a future surgical facelift.

Types of Threads Available on the Market

Thread lifts are categorized based on their composition and function:

1. Mini (Mono) Threads For Collagen Stimulation

Thin, smooth threads placed in a mesh pattern under the skin.

Do not lift but stimulate collagen production over time.

Best for improving skin texture, fine lines, and mild laxity.

Common areas: Cheeks, neck, under-eye, jawline, and decolletage.

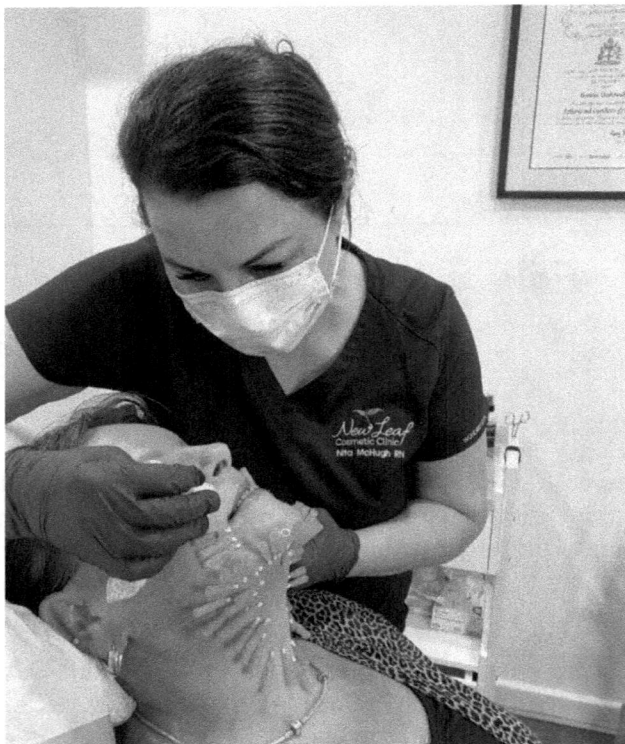

2. Cogged (Barbed) Thread: For Lifting & Contouring

Have tiny barbs/hooks that anchor into tissue, allowing mechanical lifting of sagging skin.

Best for jawline definition, mid-face lifting, and reducing jowls. Stimulate collagen as they dissolve, improving firmness and elasticity.

3. Screw & Tornado Threads For Volume Enhancement

Twisted threads that create mild volumization in areas of hollowing.

Best for nasolabial folds, cheeks, and temples.

4. PLLA & PCL Threads Longer-Lasting Bio-Stimulatory Threads

Made from poly-L-lactic acid (PLLA) or polycaprolactone (PCL), which stimulate collagen for a longer period than traditional PDO threads.

Best for long-term skin rejuvenation rather than lifting.

How Do Threads Work?

Mechanical Lift (for cogged threads) Immediate lifting effect as the barbs hook into tissue.

Collagen Stimulation (for all threads) The body responds to the threads as a foreign material, triggering fibroblast activity and new collagen synthesis.

Gradual Dissolution :Threads break down over time while leaving new collagen in place for longer-lasting effects.

Best Patient Selection for Thread Lifts

Ideal Candidates:

Mild to moderate skin laxity (not excessive sagging).

Good skin quality with some elasticity (threads work best if the skin still has some natural firmness). Patients who want a non-surgical option for lifting or rejuvenation. Those who are open to combined treatments (threads alone may not be enough for full correction).

Not Suitable For:

Severe skin laxity or heavy sagging these patients would benefit more from a facelift. Very thin, atrophic skin (threads may not hold well). Patients with active infections or autoimmune conditions affecting healing.

Threads Work Best in Combination with Fillers & Bio-Stimulants While threads provide lift and collagen stimulation, they do not restore lost volume. The best results are seen when threads are combined with dermal fillers, PRP, or bio-stimulants like Sculptra or Radiesse.

Threads + Fillers: Restores both structure and volume, preventing a flat or tightened but hollow look.

Threads + PRP/Exosomes: Enhances healing and collagen production.

Threads + Skin Boosters: Improves skin hydration and elasticity.

How Long Do Threads Last?

Immediate lifting effect : Visible right after the procedure, but best results are seen 3-6 months later due to collagen remodeling.

Longevity depends on the type of thread used:

Thread Type	Dissolution Time	Collagen Stimulation Duration
PDO (Polydioxanone)	4-6 months	Up to 12 months
PLLA (Poly-L-Lactic Acid)	12-18 months	Up to 2 years
PCL (Polycaprolactone)	18-24 months	Up to 3 years

Maintenance treatments every 12-18 months help maintain results over time.

What Happens to Threads in the Body?

Threads are absorbable .They break down naturally through hydrolysis (a process where water molecules dissolve the material). As they dissolve, the body replaces them with collagen, prolonging the skin-tightening effects. No permanent foreign material remains after full absorption.

Potential Complications of Thread Lifts

While thread lifts are generally safe, complications can occur, particularly if the procedure is performed by an inexperienced injector.

Mild Side Effects (Expected & Temporary): Swelling and bruising (common for 1-2 weeks). Mild discomfort or tightness.

Possible Risks:

Thread migration (if placed incorrectly, threads can move). Visible or palpable threads (especially in thin skin). Asymmetry if one side tightens more than the other. Dimples or puckering (usually resolves as swelling subsides).

CHAPTER 40: HOW PAINFUL ARE INJECTABLE TREATMENTS?

Pain tolerance varies from person to person, but most injectable treatments are well tolerated when performed by a skilled injector. The level of discomfort depends on the type of procedure, technique used, injection depth, and area treated. Fortunately, various pain management strategies, including numbing creams, vibration devices, ice, and anaesthetics can help minimize discomfort. This chapter breaks down the pain levels associated with different injectables and thread lifts, as well as the best methods for pain relief during treatments.

Pain Levels by Treatment Type

1. Dermal Fillers : Minimal Pain with Proper Technique

Skilled injectors can inject gently and precisely, minimizing discomfort.

Numbing cream (topical anaesthetic) is applied before treatment.

Most HA fillers contain lidocaine, which numbs the area as the injection progresses.

Pain Factors:

Needle injections can sting, especially if a blood vessel is accidentally pierced, leading to bruising and swelling.

Swelling and bruising last 1-2 weeks but are temporary.

Cannula technique is often less painful than needles but can feel uncomfortable when breaking through septa (connective tissue compartments), sometimes producing a crunchy sensation.

Pain Relief Options:

1. Topical numbing cream (BLT: Benzocaine, Lidocaine, Tetracaine) Applied 20-30 minutes before treatment.

Dental block (for lips) :Numbs the entire lip area but may cause temporary facial numbness.

Cold compress/ice :Reduces pain and swelling.

Distraction devices (e.g., squeeze balls, vibration pens) Help divert attention from discomfort.

Lips are one of the most sensitive areas, so stronger numbing options like a dental block or BLT cream are often recommended.

2. Cannula vs. Needle : Which Is More Comfortable?

Cannulas require only one or two entry points per treatment area.

Less trauma to blood vessels = fewer bruises and less swelling.

Cannula injections feel more like pressure rather than a sharp sting.

However, the cannula must break through the septa (fibrous tissue), which can feel crunchy and slightly uncomfortable.

A small amount of local anaesthetic is injected at the cannula entry point to reduce pain.

3. Botulinum Toxin (Botox, Dysport, Xeomin, etc.) Stings Slightly Botulinum toxin is mixed with saline, which can cause a mild stinging sensation.

The injections use very fine needles, but they can feel sharper as the needle blunts over multiple injections.

Pain Management:

Ice before and after can reduce discomfort.

Fast injections with minimal passes reduce needle fatigue and pain.

4. Thread Lifts Discomfort During and After

Threads are infused with lidocaine to numb the treatment area during insertion.

However, discomfort and soreness are common after the anaesthetic wears off, lasting up to a week.

Pain Management for Threads:

Oral painkillers (paracetamol, ibuprofen) can help with post-treatment soreness.

Avoid excessive movement or stretching for the first few days to minimize discomfort.

Full-face thread lifts involve multiple entry points, so post-procedure soreness is expected.

5. Nitrous Oxide (Laughing Gas) Available in Some Clinics

Nitrous oxide (laughing gas) is available in some clinics to reduce anxiety and pain.

Provides a relaxing, euphoric effect while keeping the patient conscious.

Wears off quickly, allowing patients to resume normal activities immediately.

Best for patients with low pain tolerance or anxiety about injections.

Pain Reduction Strategies for Injectables

Numbing cream (BLT) Applied before treatment to reduce surface pain.

Cold compress/Ice Numbs the area and reduces swelling.

Vibration anaesthesia devices . Divert the brain's attention from the injection pain.

Squeeze balls or stress-relief tools Provide a distraction.

Shorter, faster injection sessions :Reduce overall discomfort.

Oral pain relievers (paracetamol, ibuprofen) Taken before or after treatment for pain relief.

For patients with very low pain tolerance, discussing stronger numbing options with the injector is recommended.

Conclusion: Is It Painful?

Most injectables are well tolerated, with pain levels ranging from mild to moderate.

Proper numbing and injection techniques make the experience manageable.

Cannulas reduce bruising and pain but can feel uncomfortable when breaking through tissue.

Thread lifts involve more discomfort post-procedure, but pain can be controlled with oral painkillers.

Nitrous oxide, distraction tools, and ice help reduce anxiety and pain during procedures.

A skilled injector ensures a gentle, efficient experience, making aesthetic treatments more comfortable and accessible for all patients.

CHAPTER 41: UNDERSTANDING ANAESTHETICS IN AESTHETIC MEDICINE

Aesthetic procedures often involve some level of discomfort, and the right choice of anaesthetic can significantly improve the patient experience. This chapter covers the different types of anaesthetics used in cosmetic injectables, including topical, injectable, and inhalation options, along with nerve blocks and their applications.

1. Topical Anaesthetics:

Topical anaesthetics are commonly used to numb the skin before injectable treatments, reducing pain and discomfort.

Commercially Available Topical Anaesthetics:

Lidocaine 5% (LMX, Emla, Xylocaine gel) ~Used for numbing the skin before procedures such as lip injections, laser treatments, and microneedling.

Tetracaine ~ A more potent topical anaesthetic, often combined with lidocaine for enhanced numbing.

Benzocaine ~ Found in some over-the-counter numbing gels but less commonly used in aesthetic medicine.

Compounded Topical Anaesthetics:

Custom-blended anaesthetics are formulated by compounding pharmacies for stronger and longer-lasting numbing effects.

Lidocaine + Tetracaine (23%/7%) A powerful combination used for high-pain areas like lips and tattoo removal.

BLT Cream (Benzocaine, Lidocaine, Tetracaine) A strong numbing option often used in cosmetic clinics.

Application:

Apply 20~45 minutes before the procedure, depending on formulation.

Occlusion (covering with plastic wrap) enhances absorption.

Must be removed thoroughly before injections.

2. Injectable Anaesthetics

Injectable anaesthetics provide deeper and longer-lasting numbing, often used for nerve blocks or direct infiltration.

Common Injectable Local Anaesthetics

Lidocaine 1% or 2% ~ Most commonly used; acts within minutes and lasts 1-2 hours.

Xylocaine (Lidocaine with Epinephrine) ~The addition of epinephrine prolongs numbing and reduces bleeding.

Mepivacaine ~Similar to lidocaine but longer-lasting, sometimes preferred for nerve blocks.

Use in Aesthetics:

Added to dermal fillers (some already contain lidocaine).

Directly injected before treatments like PDO threads, minor excisions, or lip fillers for extra comfort.

Used in nerve blocks to completely anaesthetise specific areas.

Lidocaine with Epinephrine ~Caution in Cardiac Patients

Epinephrine (adrenaline) is added to lidocaine to reduce bleeding and prolong the anaesthetic effect by constricting blood vessels. However, it can cause side effects, particularly in patients with heart conditions.

Potential Side Effects:

Increased heart rate (tachycardia)

Elevated blood pressure

Anxiety or restlessness

Dizziness or palpitations

In rare cases, cardiac arrhythmias

Contraindications & Cautions:

Patients with cardiovascular disease (e.g., hypertension, arrhythmias, recent heart attack) should avoid lidocaine with epinephrine.

Patients on beta-blockers or MAO inhibitors may experience an exaggerated response to epinephrine.

In cardiac patients, consider plain lidocaine without epinephrine or using the lowest effective dose.

3. Caine Poisoning - Local Anaesthetic Toxicity

Overdosing on local anaesthetics (lidocaine, tetracaine, benzocaine) can lead to systemic toxicity, known as Local Anaesthetic Systemic Toxicity (LAST).

Symptoms to Watch For:

Mild Toxicity:

Dizziness, light-headedness

Numbness around the mouth or tongue

Ringing in the ears (tinnitus)

Blurred vision

Severe Toxicity (Emergency):

Confusion, slurred speech

Muscle twitching, tremors

Seizures

Irregular heartbeat or bradycardia (slow heart rate)

Loss of consciousness

Respiratory depression

Prevention & Management:

Dose Calculation is Key ~ Ensure the total amount injected stays within safe limits (Max safe dose: 4.5 mg/kg for plain lidocaine, 7 mg/kg with epinephrine).

Aspiration Before Injection ~Prevents accidental intravascular injection.

Emergency Protocols ~ If toxicity occurs, administer IV lipid emulsion therapy immediately and provide advanced cardiac support.

4. Nerve Blocks and Their Facial Locations

Nerve blocks involve injecting anaesthetic near specific nerves to numb a large area.

Common Nerve Blocks in Aesthetic Medicine

1. Infraorbital Nerve Block ~ Numbs the lower eyelid, upper lip, and mid-face.

2. Mental Nerve Block ~Numbs the lower lip and chin.

3. Supratrochlear & Supraorbital Nerve Blocks ~ Numbs the forehead and upper face.

4. Inferior Alveolar Nerve Block ~Used for deep numbing of the lower jaw and lips.

Benefits of Nerve Blocks:

More effective than topical anaesthetics for procedures like lip injections.

Reduces swelling and distortion caused by direct local anaesthetic infiltration.

5. Inhalation Anaesthetics

Penthrox (Methoxyflurane) -(The Green Whistle)•

An inhaled analgesic commonly used in emergency settings and minor procedures. It provides rapid pain relief without needing an IV or injection.

How does it make you feel?

Mild euphoria or lightheadedness.

Relaxed, but still conscious.

Some report dizziness or nausea in higher doses.

Longevity & Usage:

Onset within minutes.

Effects last about 30~45 minutes.

Single-use; discarded after 1 dose.

Precautions:

Avoid in patients with respiratory issues or kidney problems.

Not recommended for repeated use due to potential toxicity.

Driving After Use:

Wait at least 24 hours before driving, as it may impair reflexes and judgment.

6. Nitrous Oxide (Laughing Gas) A colourless, sweet-smelling gas used for mild sedation and pain relief. Often combined with oxygen and administered through a mask.

How does it make you feel?

Light-headed, giggly, or euphoric.

Relaxed but still responsive.

May cause dizziness or a floating sensation.

Longevity & Usage:

Rapid onset (within seconds).

Effects wear off within 5~10 minutes after stopping inhalation.

Precautions:

Avoid in patients with severe respiratory conditions or vitamin B12 deficiency.

May cause nausea in some people.

Driving After Use:

Wait at least 30 minutes to 1 hour before driving.

Effects dissipate quickly, but some may still feel slightly groggy.

Choosing the right anaesthetic depends on the procedure, pain level, and patient tolerance. A combination of topical, injectable, and inhalation options can optimise comfort while ensuring safety.

CHAPTER 42: DANGERS OF INJECTABLES: UNDERSTANDING VASCULAR OCCLUSION AND ITS RISKS

Injectable treatments such as dermal fillers can provide beautiful, natural-looking results when performed by a skilled injector. However, like any medical procedure, there are risks, with vascular occlusion (VO) being one of the most serious.

A vascular occlusion occurs when filler accidentally enters or compresses a blood vessel, blocking blood flow to the surrounding tissues. If untreated, this can lead to necrosis (tissue death) or, in rare cases, blindness.

Blindness (Rare but Serious Complication)

If filler is injected into a blood vessel that supplies the eye (such as the supratrochlear or ophthalmic artery), it can cause sudden blindness. There is no current medical treatment to reverse filler-induced blindness, making prevention and immediate action critical.

Stroke (Extremely Rare but Possible)

If filler enters the brains blood supply, it could cause neurological damage.

Signs of a Vascular Occlusion (VO)

Immediate Signs (During or Immediately After Injection):

Blanching (White or Gray Skin) " Lack of blood flow makes the skin look pale, gray, or mottled in the affected area.

No Blood Return When Pressing (Capillary Refill Delay) When pressing on the skin, it does not turn pink again within 2-3 seconds.

Sudden, Severe Pain .Patients often describe it as a burning, intense pain that worsens over time.

Cold Skin Temperature . The skin may feel unusually cold compared to surrounding areas.

Signs of Necrosis (Hours to Days After Injection):

Increasing Pain and Skin Darkening .The area may turn dusky, purple, or black as tissue begins to die.

Blistering or Ulceration . If untreated, the skin may form blisters and break down, leading to permanent scarring.

Delayed Wound Healing or Open Wounds .If tissue necrosis progresses, open wounds and deep scarring can develop.

What to Do If You Have These Signs?

1. Seek Immediate Help From Your Injector

Contact your injector IMMEDIATELY if you experience pain, blanching, or delayed capillary refill.

2. Apply a Warm Compress (NOT Ice)

Warmth helps dilate blood vessels and improve circulation.

Avoid ice, as it can further constrict blood flow.

3. Massage the Area Firmly (If Advised by a Professional)

Sometimes, gentle massage may help disperse the filler if the occlusion is caused by compression rather than direct arterial blockage.

4. Take Aspirin (If Advised by Your Practitioner)

Aspirin can thin the blood and improve circulation in partially blocked vessels. Only take if recommended by your injector.

How a Practitioner Will Treat a Vascular Occlusion

1. Hyaluronidase (Hyalase) Injections If an occlusion is caused by hyaluronic acid (HA) fillers, your practitioner will immediately inject hyaluronidase to dissolve the filler and restore blood flow.

2. High-Dose Hyaluronidase Repeated Every Hour (If Needed) The dose and frequency depend on the severity of the occlusion.

3. Nitroglycerin (GTN) Creams May be applied to help dilate blood vessels.

4. Oxygen Therapy (Hyperbaric Oxygen, If Available. Helps deliver oxygen to tissues at risk of necrosis.

5. Blood Thinners (If Necessary) Low-dose aspirin or anticoagulants may be used to improve circulation.

6. Follow-Up Monitoring :The practitioner will check the area for several days to ensure recovery and prevent long-term damage.

Preventing Vascular Occlusions : What Skilled Injectors Do

Knowledge of Facial Vascular Anatomy A skilled injector understands where major arteries are located and avoids high-risk areas.

Aspiration Before Injection Pulling back on the syringe before injecting can sometimes detect if a blood vessel has been entered.

Slow Injection Technique Injecting filler slowly reduces pressure and the risk of arterial blockage.

Using Cannulas in High-Risk Areas Cannulas reduce the risk of vascular occlusion because they bluntly push vessels aside instead of penetrating them.

Using the Correct Type of Filler Some fillers are more cohesive and less likely to spread into vessels.

Conclusion: Taking Occlusions Seriously

Vascular occlusions are rare but serious and can lead to skin necrosis or blindness if untreated.

Early signs include blanching, severe pain, and delayed capillary refill.

Immediate action is critical, including seeking an experienced injector, applying warmth, and using hyaluronidase for HA fillers.

Choosing a highly skilled, medically trained injector significantly reduces risks.

The best treatment for a vascular occlusion is prevention and early recognition. Knowing the signs can save your skin and vision.

Before photo. This client was treated with a "cheap" filler by an untrained injector. He was very lucky his vision wasn't affected. Not only was his skin scarred he was Psychology scarred by the necrotic tissue caused by an occlusion.

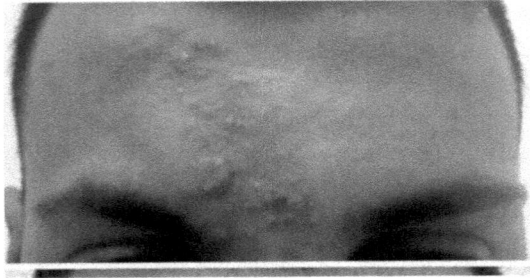

After photo: post 3 months . He was hyalased, and I treated him with Red LED sessions and a series of PRP . He healed well and luckily was not scarred .

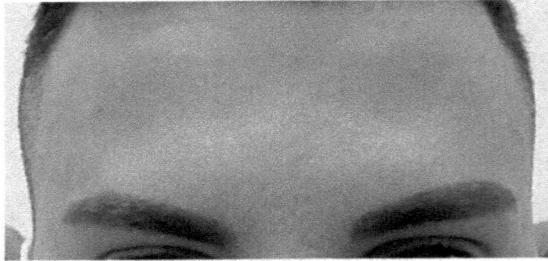

CHAPTER 43: BOTULINUM TOXIN A SIDE EFFECTS ,CAUSES, PREVENTION, AND TREATMENT

Botulinum toxin A injections (Botox, Dysport, Xeomin, Daxxify) are generally safe and well-tolerated when performed by an experienced injector. However, like any medical treatment, side effects can occur. While most are temporary, some can impact facial function and require management.

Common Botulinum Toxin A Side Effects

1. Blurred Vision & Dry Eyes

Occurs when botulinum toxin A diffuses into nearby muscles, affecting the orbicularis oculi or eye muscles responsible for blinking and tear production.

Patients may experience difficulty focusing, dry eyes, or excessive tearing.

Treatment:

Lubricating eye drops (artificial tears)

Warm compresses

Wait for botulinum toxin A to wear off (typically 4-6 weeks for mild cases)

2. Brow Ptosis (Heavy Brows or Droopy Eyebrows)

Caused by excessive botulinum toxin A in the frontalis (forehead muscle) without balancing the opposing depressor muscles.

Results in a heavy, tired-looking forehead with reduced eyebrow elevation.

Treatment:

Frown muscle (glabellar complex) botulinum toxin A can be adjusted to slightly lift the brows.

Taping techniques or facial exercises may help stimulate muscle activity.

Wait for botulinum toxin A to wear off (usually 6-8 weeks for improvement).

To avoid this: A skilled injector will ensure the correct dose and placement to maintain natural eyebrow movement.

3. Eyelid Ptosis (Drooping Eyelid)

Occurs when botulinum toxin A diffuses into the levator palpebrae muscle, which lifts the upper eyelid.

More common when treating glabellar frown lines.

Treatment:

Apraclonidine (Iopidine) 0.5% Eye Drops .Temporarily lifts the eyelid by activating Mullers muscle.

Time : The effect gradually improves over 4-6 weeks as botulinum toxin A wears off.

To avoid this: The injector should place botulinum toxin A at the correct depth and avoid excessive dosing near the upper eyelid muscles.

4. Painful Welts & Histamine Reaction

Some patients experience raised, red, itchy welts at the injection site due to a localized histamine response.

Can be mistaken for an allergic reaction but is usually mild.

Treatment:

Cold compresses

Oral antihistamines (Zyrtec, Claritin)

Topical arnica or aloe vera for soothing

If symptoms persist or worsen, seek medical advice.

5. Headaches After Botulinum Toxin A Injections

Some patients experience mild headaches after treatment, likely due to:

Temporary muscle tension changes

Needle trauma

Dehydration

Treatment:

Drink plenty of water.

Take mild pain relievers like paracetamol (acetaminophen) Avoid ibuprofen or aspirin to reduce bruising risk.

Apply a cool compress to the forehead.

Headaches usually resolve within 24-48 hours.

6. Crooked Smile or Facial Asymmetry

Can occur when botulinum toxin A affects nearby muscles unintentionally.

Most commonly happens when treating:

DAO (Depressor Anguli Oris) for downturned mouth. Can lead to an uneven smile.

Masseter injections (jaw slimming).Can cause one side of the mouth to feel weaker when smiling.

Treatment:

Massage the area to encourage muscle recovery.

Neuromodulator like botulinum toxin A can be adjusted or corrected by balancing the other side.

Effects wear off in 6-12 weeks.

7. Masseter Bulge (Uneven Jawline or Lumps After Masseter Botulinum Toxin A Injections)

In some cases, one part of the masseter muscle compensates, creating an uneven bulge or hollowing.

Happens when botulinum toxin A isn't evenly distributed or when injection sites are incorrect.

Treatment:

Follow-up botulinum toxin A injections to balance the muscle activity.

Facial exercises to strengthen the weaker side.

Massage to help smooth out the muscle contraction pattern.

To prevent this: A skilled injector will analyze facial symmetry and muscle dynamics before treatment.

8. Difficulty Smiling After Masseter Botulinum Toxin A Injections

If botulinum toxin A diffuses into the risorius muscle, patients may have trouble lifting the corners of the mouth when smiling.

The smile may feel restricted or unnatural.

Treatment:

Massage and facial exercises to encourage nerve activation.

Wait 6-8 weeks for muscle function to return.

In rare cases, a small amount of additional botulinum toxin A can be placed strategically to rebalance the movement.

How Long Do Side Effects Last?

Most botulinum toxin A side effects are temporary and resolve within weeks to a few months as the toxin naturally wears off.

Side Effect Expected Duration Treatment Options

Blurred Vision / Dry Eyes 4-6 weeks Lubricating eye drops, warm compresses

Brow Ptosis (Heavy Brows) 6-8 weeks Botulinum toxin A adjustment, brow taping

Eyelid Ptosis (Droopy Eyelid) 4-6 weeks Apraclonidine eye drops

Painful Welts / Histamine Reaction 24-48 hours Antihistamines, cold compress

Headaches 24-48 hours Hydration, paracetamol, ice packs

Crooked Smile / Facial Asymmetry 6-12 weeks Massage, follow-up adjustments

Masseter Bulge 6-12 weeks Massage, additional botulinum toxin A correction

Smiling Difficulty After Masseter Botulinum Toxin A Injections 6-8 weeks Facial exercises, time

Severe or prolonged side effects should always be evaluated by a qualified injector.

Conclusion: Are Botulinum Toxin A Side Effects Serious?

Most botulinum toxin A side effects are minor, temporary, and self-resolving. Serious complications like ptosis, asymmetry, or masseter bulging can be managed with follow-up treatments. Choosing an experienced injector reduces the risk of side effects. If side effects occur, knowing what to do can help manage them effectively. The key to a successful botulinum toxin. A experience is proper technique, patient selection, and realistic expectations.

Chapter 44: Combination and Stacked Treatments

The Secret to Natural, Long-Lasting Results

One of the biggest misconceptions in aesthetic medicine is that one treatment can fix everything.

Many patients come in asking for:

- "Just a bit of Botox"

- "One syringe of filler"

- "Something for these lines"

But the face is not made of one layer, and it does not age in one way.

Aging affects:

- Bone

- Fat pads

- Ligaments

- Skin

- Muscle movement

- Collagen quality

That's why the most natural, long-lasting results come from combination treatments—also known as stacking or layering treatments.

What Are Combination or Stacked Treatments?

Combination treatments involve using more than one type of procedure, either:

- In the same session, or

- Over a series of treatments

Each treatment targets a different layer or function of the face.

Instead of trying to fix everything with filler, we treat:

- Muscle movement

- Volume loss

- Skin quality

- Collagen stimulation

- Structural support

This creates results that are:

- More natural

- Longer lasting

- More balanced

- Harder to detect

People won't say:

"You've had filler."
They'll say:

"You look amazing. What's your secret?"

Understanding the Layers of the Face

Think of the face like a house with several levels:

The Foundation: Bone

As we age:

- Bone density decreases
- The eye sockets widen
- The jawline recedes

This causes:

- Sagging
- Hollowing
- Loss of structure

Treatment:

- Structural fillers
- Biostimulants

The Support Layer: Fat Pads and Ligaments

With time:

- Fat pads shrink or descend
- Ligaments loosen

This leads to:

- Drooping cheeks
- Nasolabial folds
- Jowls

Treatment:

- Strategic filler placement
- Biostimulators

The Movement Layer: Muscles

Repeated expressions cause:

- Frown lines
- Crow's feet
- Forehead lines

Treatment:

- Botulinum toxin

The Surface Layer: Skin

Skin changes include:

- Loss of collagen
- Dehydration
- Fine lines
- Pigmentation
- Dullness

Treatment:

- Skin boosters
- PRP
- Biostimulants
- Medical-grade skincare

Why One Treatment Alone Isn't Enough

For example:

Treating only lines with filler

This may:

- Overfill the face
- Create heaviness
- Look unnatural

Treating only with toxin

This may:

- Soften lines
- But not address volume loss or skin quality

The result may still look:

- Tired
- Flat
- Hollow

True rejuvenation requires addressing multiple layers.

The Main Treatment Categories

1. Botulinum Toxin

Targets:

- Muscle movement
- Expression lines

Benefits:

- Softens frown lines
- Reduces crow's feet
- Prevents deeper wrinkles

2. Dermal Fillers

Targets:

- Volume loss
- Structural support
- Facial contours

Benefits:

- Restores cheek volume
- Defines jawline
- Softens folds

3. Biostimulants

Examples:

- Sculptra
- Radiesse
- PRP/PRF

Targets:

- Collagen production
- Skin thickness
- Structural support over time

Benefits:

- Gradual, natural improvement
- Long-lasting results

4. Skin Boosters

Targets:

- Hydration

- Skin texture
- Fine lines

Benefits:

- Smoother skin
- Improved glow
- Better elasticity

The Stacking Approach: How It Works

Instead of doing everything in one session, treatments are often layered over time.

Step 1: Relax the muscles

Botulinum toxin:

- Softens harsh expressions
- Prevents deeper lines

Step 2: Restore structure

Filler or biostimulants:

- Replace lost volume
- Support the face

Step 3: Improve skin quality

Skin boosters or PRP:

- Improve texture
- Stimulate collagen
- Add hydration

This approach creates:

- Softer expressions

- Better structure

- Healthier skin

The result is a naturally refreshed face, not an overfilled one.

Example of a Stacked Treatment Plan

Patient in her mid-40s

Concerns:

- Tired eyes

- Drooping cheeks

- Fine lines

Month 1

- Botulinum toxin: frown, forehead, crow's feet

Month 2

- Cheek filler or biostimulant for structure

Month 3

- Skin booster or PRP for skin quality

Maintenance

- Toxin every 3–4 months

- Skin boosters twice a year

- Structural treatment every 12–24 months

This creates:

- Natural, progressive improvement

- No sudden, obvious changes

The Advantages of Combination Treatments

More Natural Results

No single area is overtreated.

Longer-Lasting Outcomes

Biostimulants and skin treatments improve collagen over time.

Better Value

Balanced treatments reduce the need for constant touch-ups.

Healthier Skin

The face looks not just fuller—but brighter and more youthful.

The Biggest Mistake: Overfilling

One of the most common problems in modern aesthetics is overuse of filler.

When filler is used to:

- Lift the face
- Improve skin quality
- Replace collagen
- Correct every line

…the result can be:

- Puffy cheeks
- Heavy faces
- Distorted proportions

This is often called:

- Pillow face
- Overfilled face
- Filler fatigue

Combination treatments reduce the need for excessive filler.

CHAPTER 45: AFTERCARE ESSENTIALS: MAXIMISE RESULTS, MINIMISE RISK

The right aftercare can make all the difference between a good result and a great one. Here's a treatment-by-treatment guide to what you should and shouldn't do after your injectable procedures.

After BOTOX/Dysport/Xeomin (Wrinkle Relaxers)

DO:

Stay upright for 4 hours

Use facial muscles (frown, smile, raise brows) to help product settle

Light walking is fine

DON'T:

No lying down or napping

Avoid strenuous exercise for 24 hours

No facial massages, saunas, or hot yoga for 48 hours

Avoid alcohol on the day of treatment

TIP: Results take 3–7 days to appear; full effect at 2 weeks.

After DERMAL FILLERS

DO:

Ice gently for 5–10 minutes at a time to reduce swelling

Sleep on your back for at least 2 nights

Keep head elevated first night

Drink plenty of water

DON'T:

No vigorous exercise for 24–48 hours

No facials or massage for 2 weeks

Don't touch, press or manipulate the area

Avoid alcohol and high-sodium foods for 24 hours

TIP: Minor swelling or bruising is common and resolves in a few days.

After SKIN BOOSTERS (e.g. Volite, NCTF 135HA)

NIGHT OF TREATMENT:

Do not apply makeup

Avoid touching or washing the area unnecessarily

Expect small papules or bumps where product was placed

NEXT DAY (AND ONWARD):

Use gentle cleanser and moisturiser

Resume makeup if no open punctures remain

Avoid harsh exfoliants or acids for 3–5 days

No sauna or vigorous exercise for 24–48 hours

TIP: Redness or papules usually subside within 24–72 hours.

After BIOSTIMULANTS (e.g. Sculptra, Lenisna, Radiesse, Juvelook)

DO:

Massage the treated areas for 5 minutes, 5 times a day, for 5 days (unless otherwise advised)

Use a clean moisturiser or oil to aid massage

Stay hydrated—biostimulants love water

DON'T:

No intense exercise or facial treatments for 1 week

Avoid alcohol, blood thinners, and anti-inflammatories for 24 hours

TIP: Collagen stimulation is gradual—results may build over 6–12 weeks and may require multiple sessions.

After PRP (Platelet-Rich Plasma)

DO:

Keep skin clean and dry for the first 12 hours

Use only gentle, non-active skincare for 2–3 days

Sleep on a clean pillowcase

DON'T:

Avoid anti-inflammatories (e.g., Nurofen, aspirin) for 5–7 days—they can blunt the healing response

No active skincare, acids, or vitamin A for 3–5 days

No makeup for 12–24 hours

Avoid sun exposure for 48 hours

TIP: Tingling, redness or pinpoint bruising is normal and settles quickly. PRP is about healing—not instant plumping.

When to ICE (and when not to)

YES—Ice After:

Filler (especially lips or tear troughs): Helps reduce swelling and bruising

Skin boosters if swollen

After any injectables to ease discomfort (short, clean applications)

NO—Do Not Ice:

After PRP: Cold suppresses inflammation, which you actually want for collagen stimulation

Over-massage or apply prolonged pressure with ice: Can worsen bruising

.

CHAPTER 46: WHAT IS DYSMORPHIA

What is Dysmorphia?

Dysmorphia, or Body Dysmorphic Disorder (BDD), is a psychological condition where a person becomes excessively preoccupied with perceived flaws in their appearance. These flaws may be minor or even non-existent, but to the individual, they feel overwhelming and distressing.

BDD is not simply about disliking certain features most people have aspects of their appearance they'd like to change. Instead, it is a persistent and obsessive concern that negatively impacts daily life, relationships, and self-esteem.

How Do You Know If You Have Dysmorphia?

If you find yourself constantly preoccupied with your appearance, it's important to ask: Is my concern reasonable, or is it taking over my thoughts and emotions?

Here are some signs that you might be experiencing Body Dysmorphic Disorder:

1. You Obsess Over a Specific Feature

You spend hours daily thinking about a perceived flaw.

You check your appearance excessively in mirrors or completely avoid them.

You take multiple photos, zooming in to analyse the feature.

2. Your Self-Worth is Tied to Your Looks

Your mood and confidence depend on how you think you look that day.

A bad appearance day can lead to anxiety, depression, or avoiding social events.

3. You Constantly Compare Yourself to Others

You feel inadequate when you see photos of others, particularly influencers or celebrities.

You frequently use filters or editing apps to create an idealized version of yourself.

4. You Seek Reassurance, but It's Never Enough

You frequently ask others if they notice your flaw or if you look okay.

Even when people reassure you, you don't believe them.

5. You Have a History of Unnecessary or Excessive Cosmetic Procedures

You have had multiple treatments but still feel dissatisfied.

You keep searching for the perfect fix, even when professionals advise against further procedures.

You feel temporary relief after a treatment, but the anxiety returns or shifts to another feature.

6. Your Daily Life is Affected

You avoid social situations because you feel too self-conscious. You spend excessive time or money on makeup, skincare, or cosmetic treatments in an attempt to fix the issue.

You feel anxious or depressed when thinking about your appearance. If you relate to several of these signs, it might indicate BDD or an unhealthy relationship with your self-image.

What Can Be Done? Treatment for Dysmorphia

Recognizing that your thoughts about your appearance may not be rational is the first step. BDD is a treatable condition, and the right approach can help you regain control over your self-image.

1. Seek Professional Help

A psychologist or therapist specializing in body image issues can help. Cognitive Behavioural Therapy (CBT) is the gold standard treatment for BDD, helping individuals challenge and reframe distorted thoughts about their appearance.

2. Reduce Mirror-Checking & Social Media Exposure

Limit time spent looking in mirrors or taking selfies. Reduce time on social media, particularly pages that promote unrealistic beauty standards.

3. Avoid Repeated Cosmetic Procedures

If you've had multiple treatments and still feel dissatisfied, further procedures are unlikely to help. Aesthetic professionals have an ethical responsibility to refuse treatments if they suspect BDD.

4. Shift the Focus to What Your Body Can Do

Instead of fixating on appearance, focus on your body's strength, health, and abilities. Engage in activities that make you feel good, like exercise, yoga, or dance, without focusing on aesthetics.

5. Practice Self-Compassion

Recognise that perfection does not exist and beauty is subjective. Learn to speak kindly to yourself, the way you would to a friend.

6. Consider Medication (If Needed)

In severe cases, SSRIs (Selective Serotonin Reuptake Inhibitors), a type of antidepressant, can help reduce obsessive thoughts. Medication should be discussed with a mental health professional.

Final Thoughts

Aesthetic treatments should enhance confidence, not fuel insecurities. If concerns about appearance start to dominate your life, it's worth reflecting on whether it's more than just dissatisfaction it could be dysmorphia.

Seeking help is not about giving up on looking good, but about achieving a healthier relationship with yourself. True beauty comes from self-acceptance, and no amount of cosmetic treatments can replace inner peace.

CHAPTER 47: HEALTH IS WEALTH

I am a great advocate for integrative medicine, recognizing that our internal health is reflected in our external appearance. The way we eat, drink, sleep, and manage stress directly influences how we look. Many aesthetic concerns are symptoms of underlying health issues, and addressing the root cause leads to lasting beauty and rejuvenation.

How Health Affects Appearance

1. Lifestyle Factors and Their Visible Impact

Alcohol Causes bloating, puffy eyes, and ruddy (red, inflamed) skin due to dehydration and liver stress.

Cigarettes Leads to poor circulation, smoker's lines, and wrinkled, grey-toned skin from oxygen deprivation.

Dehydration Results in dry, crepey skin and increased fine lines due to lack of hydration at the cellular level.

Obesity Can contribute to fuller facial features, double chins, and increased facial fat deposits, sometimes making aging signs more prominent.

2. Hormonal Health and Its Aesthetic Impact

Thyroid Issues : Hypothyroidism can cause hair loss, weight gain, and dry, flaky skin, while hyperthyroidism may lead to thin, fragile skin and excessive hair shedding.

Perimenopause & Postmenopause :The loss of oestrogen leads to skin thinning, dryness, fine lines, and loss of elasticity.

Testosterone Imbalance : Can contribute to excessive facial hair in women or hair loss on the scalp.

3. Mental Health and the Face

Depression, Anxiety & Insomnia :Poor sleep causes dark circles, fine lines, dull skin, and increased facial tension (frown lines, clenched jaw).

Anorexia & Malnutrition :Leads to severe facial fat loss, hollow cheeks, thinning hair, and dull skin due to lack of essential nutrients.

Grief and Sadness: Emotionally, sadness can be seen in the droop of the corners of the mouth, tension in the forehead, and a general loss of facial vibrancy.

4. The Role of Vitamins & Minerals in Skin Health

Vitamin C Deficiency: Causes weakened gums, dull skin, and slower collagen production.

Vitamin D Deficiency :Can lead to dull, dry skin and increased skin aging due to its role in cell turnover.

B Vitamins & the MTHFR Gene Mutation: Many people have undiagnosed MTHFR gene mutations, affecting their ability to process B vitamins, impacting oestrogen metabolism and skin quality.

Lack of Minerals (Zinc, Magnesium, Selenium, etc.) Affects immune function, skin hydration, and overall skin integrity.

5. Chronic Health Conditions and Aesthetic Changes

Stress & Cortisol Overload :Leads to premature aging, breakouts, dull skin, and deepened facial lines.

Diabetes : Can cause poor wound healing, dark patches (acanthosis nigricans), and overall dull skin tone.

Fibromyalgia: Often linked to chronic fatigue, pale skin, and premature aging signs due to persistent pain and stress.

Cosmetic Procedures & Medical Conditions

Many medical conditions affect when and how cosmetic treatments can be performed. Here are a few key considerations:

Cancer & Chemotherapy :Skin becomes fragile, and immune function is compromised. When is it safe to start cosmetic procedures post-treatment? It's usually recommended to wait at least 6-12 months post-chemo and only proceed under medical guidance.

Acne & Roaccutane (Isotretinoin): Patients on Roaccutane should avoid laser treatments and deep peels as the skin is highly sensitive and prone to scarring. Treatments should resume 6 months post-medication.

Herpes Simplex (Cold Sores) : Cosmetic treatments like lip fillers or microneedling can trigger outbreaks. Pre-treatment antiviral medication (e.g., Valacyclovir) is recommended to prevent post-procedure flare-ups.

Final Thoughts: A Holistic Approach to Beauty

True rejuvenation is not just about injectables and skin treatments it's about nourishing the body, balancing hormones, managing stress, and understanding the deep connection between health and beauty.

Rather than masking symptoms, I believe in addressing the root cause, helping individuals heal from within so their outer beauty naturally radiates vitality and wellness. Because at the end of the day, health truly is wealth.

CHAPTER 48: THE MOST IMPORTANT BEAUTY TREATMENT IS FREE!

Water: The Ultimate Beauty Secret

In my opinion, the most essential beauty treatment doesn't cost a cent it Is water! Hydration is the foundation of good skin, internal health, and overall well-being. While people chase the latest skincare trends and cosmetic treatments, many overlook the simplest, most powerful anti-aging tool is proper hydration.

What Does Water Do for Your Skin and Body?

1. Water & The Skin

Hydrated skin appears plumper, smoother, and more radiant.

Dehydrated skin looks dull, wrinkled, and tired, often with more pronounced fine lines.

Reduces dryness and flakiness, improving skin texture.

Flushes toxins that contribute to breakouts and inflammation.

Helps prevent premature aging by maintaining skin elasticity.

2. Water & The Liver

The liver is the body's natural detoxifier. Water helps flush out toxins, preventing congestion that can lead to dull skin, acne, and inflammation.

Proper hydration reduces dark circles and puffiness, which are often signs of liver stress and poor circulation.

3. Water & The Bowels

Hydration is key to regular bowel movements. When we are dehydrated, our digestive system slows down, leading to constipation and bloating.

Regular bowel movements prevent toxin buildup, which can contribute to skin congestion and breakouts.

My Morning Hydration Ritual

Every morning, before coffee or tea, I drink an entire litre of water is a non-negotiable part of my beauty routine.

Why?

We lose water while we sleep, leading to morning dehydration.

Drinking water first thing helps flush toxins, rehydrate the body, and wake up the digestive system.

It gets the bowels moving, ensuring regular elimination.

It prevents headaches most headaches are due to dehydration!

It hydrates the brain, helping with mental clarity and focus.

Coffee and tea are diuretics, which means they can contribute to dehydration if consumed first thing.

Hydrated Skin vs. Dehydrated Skin: The Visible Difference

Hydrated Skin:

Glows naturally

Looks plump and youthful

Has fewer visible fine lines

Feels smooth and supple

Dehydrated Skin:

Looks dull and tired

Shows fine lines and wrinkles more prominently

Appears rough and flaky

Can look puffy yet dry at the same time

Water & The Kidneys: Say Goodbye to Dark Circles

Dark circles aren't t always from lack of sleep they can also be a sign of dehydration and poor kidney function. Drinking enough water helps flush the kidneys, reducing the appearance of dark circles and under-eye puffiness.

Final Thoughts: The Simplest Beauty Hack

Before you spend hundreds on skincare and treatments, ask yourself-are you drinking enough water? Good hydration is the most overlooked yet powerful beauty treatment. It benefits your skin, digestion, energy, and overall health and best of all, it is completely free.

Start your day with water.

Drink 2-3 litres a day and your body and skin will thank you.

CHAPTER 49: ANTI-AGING TRENDS

Aging gracefully is no longer just about skincare and injectables scientific advancements in longevity and regenerative medicine are revolutionizing the way we approach aging. From IV infusions to peptide therapy, cutting-edge treatments are emerging that focus on cellular health, hormone balance, and mitochondrial function.

Here are some of the latest anti-aging trends that are shaping the future of longevity.

1. IV Infusions: Replenishing from the Inside Out

Intravenous (IV) therapy delivers vitamins, minerals, antioxidants, and hydration directly into the bloodstream, bypassing the digestive system for maximum absorption.

Popular IV infusions for anti-aging include:

Glutathione: A powerful antioxidant that brightens skin, detoxifies the liver, and reduces oxidative stress.

Vitamin C: Boosts collagen production and immunity.

B Vitamins: Essential for energy, metabolism, and brain function.

NAD+ (Nicotinamide Adenine Dinucleotide): A game-changer in longevity science.

2. NAD+ Therapy: Cellular Energy & DNA Repair

NAD+ is a coenzyme found in every cell that plays a critical role in energy production and DNA repair. As we age, NAD+ levels decline, leading to fatigue, inflammation, and slower cellular repair.

NAD+ infusions or supplements (like NMN and NR) help to:

Improve mitochondrial function (the powerhouse of cells).

Increase energy and cognitive function.

Slow down aging at the cellular level.

NMN (Nicotinamide Mononucleotide) & NR (Nicotinamide Riboside):

These precursors to NAD+ boost cellular metabolism and longevity.

Studies suggest they may delay age-related diseases and improve skin health.

3. Low Dose Naltrexone (LDN): Inflammation & Immune Support

LDN, originally used to treat opioid addiction, is now being studied for its ability to regulate the immune system and reduce chronic inflammation a key driver of aging.

Potential anti-aging benefits of LDN:

Reduces chronic inflammation, which contributes to aging and disease.

May help with autoimmune conditions, fibromyalgia, and chronic pain.

Can improve sleep and mood, essential for longevity.

4. Transdermal Hormones: Balancing the Aging Body

Hormonal imbalances contribute to skin aging, weight gain, fatigue, and cognitive decline. Instead of oral hormone replacement, transdermal (topical) hormone therapy is gaining popularity due to its better absorption and lower risk of liver stress.

Key anti-aging hormones include:

Oestrogen (Bioidentical HRT) Maintains skin elasticity, prevents bone loss, and supports cognitive function.

Testosterone:(for men and women) Preserves muscle mass, libido, and mental clarity.

Progesterone: Regulates mood, sleep, and inflammation.

DHEA & Pregnenolone: Anti-aging hormones that support energy, cognition, and immune function.

5. X39 Stem Cell Activation Patches

The X39 patch is a light-activated therapy that claims to stimulate the body's natural production of stem cells-a key factor in tissue repair and longevity.

Reported benefits include:

Improved wound healing and skin rejuvenation.

Increased energy and mental clarity.

Faster muscle recovery and reduced inflammation.

6. PEMF Mats: Electromagnetic Healing

Pulsed Electromagnetic Field (PEMF) therapy uses low-frequency electromagnetic waves to stimulate cellular repair, reduce inflammation, and enhance circulation.

Anti-aging benefits of PEMF therapy:

Improves sleep and cellular regeneration.

Reduces pain and inflammation.

Supports bone density and joint health.

Enhances mitochondrial function, slowing cellular aging.

7. Amino Acids for Muscle Preservation & Longevity

Muscle loss (sarcopenia) is a major concern with aging, affecting metabolism, strength, and skin integrity. Amino acids play a crucial role in muscle maintenance, collagen production, and energy metabolism.

Key amino acids for anti-aging:

L-Glutamine: Supports gut health, muscle recovery, and immune function.

L-Carnitine: Aids in fat metabolism and energy production.

Collagen Peptides: Boost skin elasticity, hair health, and joint function.

BCAAs (Branched-Chain Amino Acids): Preserve muscle mass and improve endurance.

8. Other Cutting-Edge Anti-Aging Trends

Peptides & Growth Factors

GHK-Cu (Copper Peptide): Known for its skin regeneration and wound healing properties.

Epitalon: A longevity peptide that may extend lifespan by regulating telomere length.

Thymosin Beta-4: Promotes tissue repair and reduces inflammation.

Cold Therapy (Cryotherapy & Ice Baths)

Reduces inflammation and oxidative stress.

Enhances circulation and fat metabolism.

Increases endorphins and energy levels.

Red Light Therapy (Photobiomodulation)

Stimulates collagen production and improves skin texture.

Enhances cellular energy (ATP production).

Helps with wound healing, hair growth, and pain relief.

Fasting & Autophagy

Intermittent fasting and prolonged fasting trigger autophagy, the body's natural process of removing damaged cells and regenerating new ones. Fasting is linked to increased longevity, reduced inflammation, and improved metabolic health.

Peptides: What They Are and Why Everyone Is Talking About Them

A peptide is a short chain of amino acids (the building blocks of protein). You can think of peptides as biological "messengers". In the body, different peptides signal different actions — such as inflammation control, tissue repair, pigmentation, growth hormone signalling, immune modulation, or sleep–wake rhythm regulation.

In aesthetics and longevity medicine, peptides are popular because they're marketed as "targeted" and "natural," with claims around skin quality, healing, fat loss, energy, sleep, and healthy ageing. However, the science and regulation are mixed: some peptides are legitimate medicines, while others are experimental or unapproved.

The Anti-Ageing Peptide Trend

Peptides sit at the intersection of three booming trends:

Longevity medicine (optimising sleep, recovery, inflammation, metabolic health)

Regenerative aesthetics (skin quality, collagen support, wound healing)

Biohacking culture (self-experimentation, online peptide "stacks")

This has created a fast-moving market where marketing often runs ahead of evidence. A key message for consumers is this:

Not all peptides are equal. Some have solid medical uses. Others have early research only. Some sold online are poor quality, incorrectly dosed, or not what they claim.

Common Peptides People Ask About (and What They're Promoted For)

Skin and collagen support

GHK-Cu (Copper peptide)

Most commonly used topically in skincare

Promoted for skin repair and collagen support

Topical cosmetic products are widely available; injectable forms raise bigger safety and regulatory issues

Longevity and sleep rhythm

Epithalon (Epitalon / Epithalamin)

A short synthetic peptide linked to the pineal gland and circadian rhythm research

Promoted for sleep quality, "longevity," and cellular ageing support

Evidence is limited and it is not a mainstream approved medicine in Australia.

Healing and tissue repair (popular online, high caution)

BPC-157 and TB-500 / Thymosin beta fragments

Promoted for tendon, ligament, gut repair, and injury recovery

Much of the hype is based on preclinical or early research and heavy online marketing

This is one of the most common areas where people buy unsafe "research peptides" online

Immune and inflammation support (medical-adjacent use)

Thymosin Alpha-1 (TA1)

Studied for immune modulation

In some countries used in specific medical contexts

Access and appropriateness depend entirely on medical oversight and local regulation

Pigmentation (not "anti-ageing," but common in aesthetics circles)

Melanotan

Promoted for tanning and sometimes appetite/sexual effects

Higher risk profile, commonly sourced illegally, and not something I recommend

Important note for readers: many peptide claims are off-label or not proven, and results vary widely.

Where to Get Peptides Safely (Australia)

In Australia, many peptides discussed online are not on the ARTG (not approved/registered for general supply). When a product is "unapproved," legal access may still be possible through the correct medical pathways.

1) Through a registered medical practitioner using TGA pathways

The TGA allows access to unapproved therapeutic goods via the Special Access Scheme (SAS) and other pathways, where a practitioner applies or notifies for a specific patient and clinical need.

2) Via legitimate pharmacy compounding (prescription only)

Some medicines can be compounded for an individual patient when clinically appropriate. Compounding is governed by professional standards and quality expectations, and it is not meant to be "mass produced" or casually supplied.

3) Clinical trials

For emerging therapies, clinical trials are often the safest and most transparent access route.

The big red flag

If someone is selling peptides directly to the public online, especially labelled "research use only," that is a major safety risk. Purity, sterility, and dosing accuracy can be unreliable.

Final Thoughts: The Future of Anti-Aging

We are entering an exciting era of longevity science, where the focus is shifting from just treating aging signs externally to optimizing health at a cellular level. While injectables and skincare remain valuable tools, true anti-aging goes far beyond aesthetics "it is about extending vitality, cognitive function, and overall quality of life.

From IV infusions and NAD+ therapy to hormonal balance, peptides, and biohacking, the future of aging gracefully is about integrative, regenerative, and preventive medicine.

The goal? Not just to look younger but to feel stronger, sharper, and healthier for years to come.

CHAPTER 50: BEAUTY STARTS IN THE GUT

They say beauty comes from within, and in many ways, that starts with the gut. The health of our gut microbiome directly impacts our skin, hair, energy levels, and overall well-being. Many people focus on external beauty treatments without realizing that poor gut health can manifest as skin issues, inflammation, and premature aging.

How Today's Diet Harms the Gut

Our modern lifestyle has disrupted gut health, leading to an imbalance in the gut microbiome (dysbiosis). Some of the biggest offenders include:

Antibiotics in Food: Wipe out both good and bad bacteria, leading to an unhealthy microbiome.

Too Much Gluten: Can trigger gut inflammation and leaky gut syndrome, especially in sensitive individuals.

Excess Sugar: Feeds bad bacteria and yeast (candida), contributing to acne, dull skin, and bloating.

Too Much Lactose (Dairy Products) Dairy intolerance can cause skin breakouts, puffiness, and digestive discomfort.

Gut Imbalance & Beauty Problems

When the gut microbiome is imbalanced, it can show up in various beauty concerns:

Acne: Overgrowth of bad bacteria and candida can cause hormonal imbalances, inflammation, and breakouts.

Eczema & Rosacea: Linked to leaky gut and inflammation.

Dull, Dry Skin: Poor gut health reduces nutrient absorption, leading to lacklustre skin.

Dark Circles & Puffiness: Toxins from gut imbalances burden the liver and kidneys, causing fluid retention and dark under-eye circles.

Thinning Hair: Nutrient deficiencies from poor digestion impact hair growth and scalp health.

How to Repair Leaky Gut

A damaged gut lining (leaky gut) allows toxins and undigested food particles to enter the bloodstream, triggering inflammation, autoimmune reactions, and skin conditions. Here's how to heal it:

1. Nutrients & Supplements for Gut Repair

Butyric Acid: A short-chain fatty acid that helps heal the gut lining and reduce inflammation.

Glutathione: A powerful antioxidant that supports liver detoxification and gut barrier integrity.

Berberine: A natural antibacterial that reduces bad bacteria overgrowth and improves insulin sensitivity.

Oregano Oil: Helps eliminate harmful bacteria, parasites, and candida overgrowth.

Slippery Elm: Soothes and coats the gut lining, reducing inflammation.

Triphala: An Ayurvedic herbal blend that supports digestion and detoxification.

Water: Hydration is essential for flushing out toxins and supporting digestive function.

2. Reduce Foods That Trigger Inflammation

To heal the gut, it is essential to remove inflammatory foods, including:

Refined Sugar (feeds bad bacteria and candida).

Processed Foods & Artificial Additives (disrupt microbiome balance).

Excessive Gluten & Dairy (can trigger inflammation in sensitive individuals).

3. Support Digestion & Reduce Bloating

Many people lack digestive enzymes, leading to poor breakdown of foods like red meat and lectins (found in legumes, grains, and nightshades). When undigested food sits in the small intestine, it can cause bacterial overgrowth, bloating, gas, and puffiness.

Digestive Enzymes: Help break down food properly, preventing gut irritation.

Probiotics & Prebiotics: Balance good bacteria for better digestion and skin health.

Fermented Foods: (Kimchi, sauerkraut, kefir) naturally restore gut microbiome balance.

Testing for Gut Health

For those experiencing chronic skin issues, bloating, fatigue, or food intolerances, it is beneficial to see an integrative doctor to analyse stool samples for gut bacteria levels, yeast overgrowth, and markers of inflammation.

The Effects of Candida Overgrowth on Skin & Beauty

Candida (a type of yeast) is naturally present in the body, but excess sugar, antibiotics, and stress can cause it to overgrow. When candida takes over, it can wreak havoc on the skin.

Common Symptoms of Candida Overgrowth:

Persistent acne, rashes, or fungal skin infections.

White coating on the tongue (oral thrush).

Digestive issues like bloating, gas, and sugar cravings.

Chronic fatigue and brain fog.

How to Treat Candida Naturally:

Cut out sugar & refined carbs (which feed candida).

Increase probiotics to restore gut balance.

Use natural antifungals like oregano oil, berberine, and caprylic acid.

Aloe Vera: A Superfood for Gut & Skin

Aloe vera isn't just for soothing sunburns it is a powerful gut healer!

Aloe Vera Benefits for the Gut:

Soothes and repairs the gut lining.

Supports healthy digestion and reduces bloating.

Helps balance gut bacteria.

Aloe Vera Benefits for Skin:

Hydrates and calms inflammation.

Contains vitamins and antioxidants that boost collagen production.

Supports wound healing and reduces acne scars.

Drinking aloe vera juice (with no added sugar) can be a great way to support gut and skin health simultaneously.

Final Thoughts: Gut Health is the Foundation of Beauty

The gut-skin connection is undeniable. Many common skin issues are rooted in poor digestion, microbiome imbalances, and leaky gut.

By healing the gut with the right foods, supplements, and lifestyle changes, we can achieve clearer skin, stronger hair, reduced inflammation, and a more radiant complexion true beauty from the inside out.

CHAPTER 51: THYROID HEALTH AND ITS IMPACT ON FACIAL APPEARANCE

When discussing beauty and rejuvenation, it's essential to start with the foundations of health. One of the most overlooked contributors to facial puffiness, tired appearance, and skin texture changes is thyroid dysfunction—specifically hypothyroidism. The thyroid gland plays a crucial role in regulating metabolism, energy production, and cellular repair. When the thyroid is underactive (hypothyroidism), the entire body slows down, and the face often provides early visual clues that something is not functioning optimally.

Common Symptoms of Hypothyroidism

Persistent fatigue

Weight gain, even with unchanged diet and exercise habits

Dry skin

Feeling cold easily

Depression or low mood

Constipation

Hair thinning, particularly the outer third of the eyebrows

Puffy face and eyelids

Hoarseness of voice

Slowed heart rate

From an aesthetic viewpoint, two signs are particularly notable:

Puffiness of the face, especially around the eyes and jawline.

Thinning of the lateral (outer) third of the eyebrows, a classic feature often missed unless specifically looked for.

These subtle changes can make a face appear older, tired, or heavier, even if no other signs of aging are present.

Thyroid Testing and the T3 / Reverse T3 Trap

Routine thyroid tests often measure TSH (thyroid-stimulating hormone) and T4 (thyroxine). In many cases, these results may come back as "normal," leading patients to be told that their thyroid is functioning properly.

However, many symptoms can still persist despite "normal" blood tests.

This can happen when the active form of thyroid hormone, T3 (triiodothyronine), is not adequately available at the cellular level.

Even if T4 levels are normal, if the body is converting T4 into an inactive form called Reverse T3 (rT3) rather than into active T3, the cells are essentially starved of functional thyroid hormone.

This is why patients may continue to experience hypothyroid symptoms despite being prescribed thyroxine (T4 replacement therapy).

One crucial factor in this conversion process is iodine. Adequate iodine levels are needed to ensure that T4 is properly converted into bioavailable T3 rather than rT3.

What to Do if Symptoms Persist

If you or your clients are noticing ongoing symptoms of hypothyroidism — puffiness, facial swelling, thinning of the brows, or sluggishness — despite being on thyroid medication, it's important to:

See a doctor knowledgeable about full thyroid panels An integrative medicine Dr.

Request testing for Reverse T3 (rT3) and Free T3 levels

Assess iodine status if appropriate

Addressing these imbalances can significantly improve not only energy, mood, and overall health but also enhance the appearance of the face—reducing puffiness and helping to restore natural vibrancy.

Beauty Begins with Health

True aesthetic rejuvenation begins from within.

No injectable, filler, or laser can mask the signs of an underlying health issue like hypothyroidism.

As aesthetic practitioners, it's important to recognize these signs and, where appropriate, suggest medical evaluation to ensure the best long-term outcomes for clients.

A healthy thyroid often means a brighter, less puffy, more youthful appearance—naturally.

Chapter 52: Sugar: The Enemy!

In the pursuit of youthful, radiant skin, one of the most insidious adversaries is sugar. While its sweet allure is hard to resist, excessive sugar consumption wreaks havoc not only on our internal health but also on our external appearance.

The Hidden Dangers of Excess Sugar

1. Hidden Sugars in Processed Foods

Modern diets are laden with hidden sugars, often concealed under names like high fructose corn syrup, sucrose, dextrose, and more. These sugars are prevalent in processed foods, making it easy to consume excessive amounts unknowingly.

2. The Addictive Nature of Sugar

Sugar triggers the release of dopamine in the brain, creating feelings of pleasure and reward. This response can lead to cravings and overconsumption, similar to addictive substances.

Sugar's Impact on Skin Health

1. Glycation: The Silent Skin Agitator

Glycation is a natural process where excess sugar molecules bind to proteins like collagen and elastin, forming harmful compounds known as Advanced Glycation End Products (AGEs). This process compromises the integrity of these proteins, leading to:

Loss of Skin Elasticity: Skin becomes less firm and more prone to sagging.

Formation of Wrinkles: The structural damage accelerates the appearance of fine lines and wrinkles.

Dullness and Discoloration: AGEs can cause the skin to appear dull and uneven in tone.

Elevated blood sugar directly catalyzes glycation, leading to the formation of AGEs that compromise skin structure.

2. Overgrowth of Candida

Excessive sugar intake can promote the overgrowth of Candida, a type of yeast that naturally resides in the body. When Candida proliferates beyond normal levels, it can lead to:

Skin Issues: Such as fungal infections, rashes, and exacerbation of conditions like eczema.

Digestive Problems: Including bloating, gas, and discomfort.

Fatigue and Brain Fog: General feelings of tiredness and cognitive difficulties.

3. Weight Gain and Empty Calories

Sugary foods are often high in calories but low in essential nutrients, leading to weight gain and nutritional deficiencies. This not only affects overall health but also contributes to:

Increased Fat Deposits: Particularly in areas like the face and neck, affecting facial contours.

Inflammation: Which can exacerbate skin conditions like acne and rosacea.

Combating Glycation: Skin Treatments and Lifestyle Changes

While preventing glycation is ideal, certain treatments can help mitigate its effects:

1. Chemical Peels

Chemical peels involve applying a solution to the skin that exfoliates the top layers, promoting the growth of new, healthier skin. This process can improve skin texture, tone, and reduce the appearance of fine lines.

2. Laser Treatments

Laser therapies, such as fractional laser resurfacing, target deeper skin layers to stimulate collagen production and break down AGEs. This can lead to firmer, more youthful-looking skin.

3. Cosmeceuticals

Topical products containing ingredients like retinoids, antioxidants (e.g., vitamin C), and peptides can help repair and protect the skin from glycation damage. These ingredients promote collagen synthesis and neutralize free radicals.

Preventive Measures

To minimize glycation and its detrimental effects on the skin:

Limit Sugar Intake: Be mindful of both obvious and hidden sugars in your diet.

Maintain a Balanced Diet: Focus on whole foods rich in antioxidants, which combat oxidative stress and support skin health.

Stay Hydrated: Adequate water intake helps flush out toxins and supports overall skin vitality.

Sun Protection: UV exposure can exacerbate glycation; using sunscreen daily can help protect your skin.

By understanding the profound impact of sugar on our skin and overall health, we can make informed choices to preserve our natural beauty and well-being.

CHAPTER 53: GENITAL REJUVENATION WITH PLATELET-RICH PLASMA (PRP)

Platelet-Rich Plasma (PRP) therapy has emerged as a promising non-surgical option for genital rejuvenation in both men and women. By utilizing the body's own healing mechanisms, PRP aims to enhance the appearance and function of genital tissues.

PRP for Female Genital Rejuvenation

In women, PRP injections target the vulvar and vaginal areas to address various concerns:

Enhanced Appearance: PRP can improve skin texture and elasticity, leading to a more youthful vulvar appearance.

Improved Function: Benefits may include increased lubrication, heightened sensitivity, and enhanced sexual satisfaction.

Treatment of Conditions: PRP has been explored for managing symptoms of vaginal atrophy, laxity, and lichen sclerosis a condition causing thin, patchy skin in the genital area.

PRP for Male Genital Rejuvenation

For men, PRP therapy focuses on penile enhancement and addressing erectile dysfunction (ED):

Revascularization: PRP promotes the formation of new blood vessels, potentially improving blood flow to the penis, which is crucial for erectile function.

Enhanced Sensation and Performance: Men may experience increased sensitivity and improved sexual performance following PRP treatments.

The PRP Injection Procedure

The PRP treatment process is straightforward and minimally invasive:

1. **Blood Collection**: A small amount of the patient's blood is drawn.

2. **PRP Preparation**: The blood is processed in a centrifuge to concentrate the platelets, resulting in PRP rich in growth factors.

3. **Application**: The PRP is injected into specific areas of the genitalia, depending on the desired outcomes.

To minimize discomfort during the procedure, a topical anaesthetic cream, such as BLT (Benzocaine, Lidocaine, Tetracaine) cream, is applied to the treatment area prior to injection.

Treatment Frequency and Onset of Effects

Number of Treatments: Protocols vary, but a common approach involves multiple sessions. For instance, in treating female sexual dysfunction, 2 mL of PRP may be injected into the distal anterior vaginal wall once a month for three months.

Time to Notice Effects: Patients may begin to observe improvements within a few weeks after the initial treatment, with optimal results typically developing over several months.

Safety and Considerations

PRP therapy utilizes the patient's own blood components, reducing the risk of allergic reactions or rejection. However, as with any medical procedure, it's essential to consult with a qualified healthcare provider to determine if PRP is appropriate for your specific needs and to understand the potential risks and benefits involved.

By harnessing the body's natural healing processes, PRP offers a promising avenue for those seeking genital rejuvenation, aiming to enhance both aesthetic and functional aspects of the genitalia.

CHAPTER 54: MENOPAUSE

Menopause is a profound transition, not just internally but visibly on the skin and body. The hormonal shifts that occur—primarily the decline in oestrogen and progesterone—directly impact collagen levels, fat distribution, and skin hydration. This chapter explores the biological, aesthetic, and medical approaches to addressing these changes, ensuring a smoother transition into the next phase of life with confidence and vitality.

1. The Biological Impact of Menopause on the Face & Body

Hormonal Decline & Its Effect on the Skin

• **Loss of Collagen & Elasticity** → Sagging, fine lines, deeper wrinkles

• **Reduction in Skin Hydration** → Dryness, crepey texture

• **Thinning of the Epidermis** → Increased sensitivity and slower healing

• **Fat Redistribution** → Loss of facial volume, while fat accumulates in the midsection

Fat Distribution & Body Shape Changes

• **Midriff Weight Gain** → Due to declining oestrogen levels, fat shifts from hips and thighs to the abdomen

• **Loss of Muscle Mass** → Slower metabolism, contributing to stubborn fat deposits

2. Medical & Hormonal Treatments

Hormone Blood Tests & Bioidentical Hormone Therapy (BHRT)

- **Blood Tests** to assess levels of oestrogen, progesterone, testosterone, and DHEA

- **Bioidentical Hormones** (BHRT) can restore lost oestrogen, improving skin texture, hydration, and overall well-being

- **Testosterone & DHEA**: Can support muscle tone, skin thickness, and libido

Oestrogen for the Skin

- **Topical Oestrogen Creams**: Improve hydration, elasticity, and overall radiance

- **Oral or Patch Oestrogen Therapy**: Helps with systemic symptoms (hot flashes, bone density, mood) while supporting skin structure

- **Collagen Stimulation via Hormone Support**: Oestrogen encourages fibroblasts to produce more collagen, slowing down the aging process

3. Aesthetic Treatments for Menopausal Skin

Facial Treatments: Rejuvenation & Volume Restoration

Collagen Biostimulators – Sculptra, Radiesse, and PRP (Platelet-Rich Plasma) help rebuild lost collagen

Hyaluronic Acid Fillers – Restore volume loss in the mid-face, lips, and temples

Skin Boosters & Hydration Fillers – Profhilo, Juvederm Volite, or Teosyal Redensity to deeply hydrate the skin

Neuromodulators (Botox, Dysport) – Soften expression lines and prevent further deepening of wrinkles

Radiofrequency (RF) & Ultrasound Treatments (Ultherapy, Morpheus8) – Tighten sagging skin non-surgically

Chemical Peels & Laser Resurfacing – Improve skin texture, pigmentation, and elasticity

Daily Skincare Routine for Menopausal Skin

• **Retinol or Prescription Tretinoin** – Stimulates skin renewal

• **Vitamin C & Antioxidants** – Brighten skin and combat oxidative stress

• **Hyaluronic Acid & Peptides** – Maintain hydration and plumpness

• **SPF 50+ Sunscreen** – Prevents further collagen degradation

4. Addressing the Body: Fat Redistribution & Contouring

Stubborn Midriff Fat: Aesthetic & Surgical Solutions

As menopause causes fat accumulation around the midsection, diet and exercise may not be enough. The following treatments help contour the body:

Liposculpture & Liposuction

• Targets stubborn fat in the abdomen, waist, and back

• Can be combined with fat transfer to restore lost volume in the face or hands

Non-Surgical Fat Reduction

• **Cryolipolysis (CoolSculpting)** – Freezes fat cells, gradually eliminating them

• **Radiofrequency (Vanquish, TruSculpt, Exilis)** – Uses heat to shrink fat and tighten skin

Skin Tightening for the Body

• **RF Microneedling (Morpheus8 Body, Renuvion)** – Tightens loose skin and improves texture

• **HIFU (High-Intensity Focused Ultrasound)** – Non-invasive lifting for areas like the arms, abdomen, and thighs

5. Lifestyle, Nutrition & Supplement Support

Key Nutrients for Menopausal Skin & Body

• **Collagen Peptides** – Maintain skin elasticity and firmness

• **Omega-3 Fatty Acids** – Combat inflammation and dryness

• **Magnesium & Vitamin D** – Support muscle function and mood

• **Phytoestrogens (Soy, Flaxseed)** – May help balance declining oestrogen

Exercise & Body Composition

• **Strength Training** – Helps counteract muscle loss and reshape the body

• **Pilates & Yoga** – Improves posture, flexibility, and stress levels

• **Cardio Workouts** – Helps manage weight and support heart health

Conclusion: Embracing Menopause with Confidence

Menopause doesn't mean surrendering to aging—it's an opportunity to take charge of your health, appearance, and well-being. With hormonal support, aesthetic treatments, and lifestyle adjustments, you can age beautifully, naturally, and vibrantly.

CHAPTER 55: OZEMPIC FACE

Ozempic (semaglutide) and similar GLP-1 receptor agonists (e.g., Wegovy, Mounjaro) have revolutionized weight loss, helping thousands shed stubborn fat. However, rapid weight loss can have visible effects on the face, leading to a phenomenon known as "Ozempic Face."

This chapter explores the science behind facial fat loss, the specific fat pads affected, and how aesthetic treatments can restore a natural, youthful look.

What Is Ozempic Face?

How Weight Loss Affects the Face

• **Fat Redistribution & Volume Loss**: Semaglutide-induced weight loss does not discriminate—it reduces fat in the face just as it does in the body.

• **Structural Support Weakens**: With reduced deep and superficial fat pads, the face appears gaunt, hollow, and aged.

• **Skin Laxity Increases**: Without the underlying fat to "hold up" the skin, the face can appear saggy and deflated.

Common Symptoms of Ozempic Face

Hollowed cheeks

Sunken temples

More prominent nasolabial folds

Drooping jowls & marionette lines

Loose, crepey skin due to reduced elasticity

Which Facial Fat Pads Deplete?

Facial aging occurs in layers, and weight loss accelerates fat depletion in both superficial and deep fat pads.

Key Fat Pads Affected in Ozempic Face:

Fat Pad	Effect of Fat Loss
Buccal Fat Pad (Cheeks)	Sunken cheeks, gaunt appearance
Lateral Cheek Fat Pads	Loss of mid-face support, sagging
Temple Fat Pads	Hollow temples, skeletal look
Prezygomatic (Upper Cheek) Fat Pads	Loss of cheekbone definition
Submalar Fat Pads	Prominent nasolabial folds, deeper smile lines
Jawline & Submental Fat	Jowling and loose skin under the chin

Rapid weight loss can also accelerate skin aging by depleting collagen and elastin, causing wrinkles and fine lines to appear more pronounced.

How to Restore Facial Volume & Structure

Collagen Biostimulators (Sculptra & Radiesse)

Best for: Global facial rejuvenation, natural volume restoration, collagen stimulation

Sculptra (Poly-L-Lactic Acid)

• Works by stimulating collagen production over time

• Provides a gradual thickening of the skin & volume replacement

• Ideal for cheeks, temples, jawline, and overall face rejuvenation

• Results last 2+ years

Radiesse (Calcium Hydroxylapatite – CaHA)

• Provides instant volume and long-term collagen stimulation

• Great for midface, jawline, and lower face definition

• Can be used in hyperdiluted form for skin tightening

Hyaluronic Acid Fillers (HA Fillers)

Best for: Immediate volume restoration, targeted fat pad replenishment

1. Cheeks & Midface – Restores lift and support

• Juvederm Voluma, Restylane Lyft, RHA4

2. Temples – Corrects hollowing and skeletal look

• Juvederm Voluma, Restylane Lyft

3. Nasolabial Folds & Marionette Lines – Softens deep creases

• Restylane Defyne, Juvederm Ultra Plus

4. Jawline Contouring – Defines and sharpens the jawline

• Juvederm Volux, Restylane Contour

Immediate improvement with HA fillers

Lasts 12-24 months depending on the product

Skin Tightening & Regenerative Treatments

If weight loss has caused loose, sagging skin, combining volume restoration with skin-tightening therapies enhances results:

1. Radiofrequency Microneedling (Morpheus8, Profound RF) – Tightens skin, improves collagen production

2. Ultrasound (Ultherapy, Sofwave) – Lifts and firms without adding volume

3. PRP (Platelet-Rich Plasma) & Exosomes – Boosts skin regeneration and elasticity

Maintaining a Youthful Look After Weight Loss

Hydrate & Support Skin Health

• Collagen supplements (marine collagen, peptides)

• Hyaluronic acid-based skincare (topical & ingestible)

• Vitamin C & Retinol for skin renewal

Regular Aesthetic Maintenance

- Touch-ups every 12-24 months

- Non-invasive treatments to preserve elasticity & collagen

Balanced Weight Loss & Nutrition

- Losing weight gradually prevents extreme facial volume loss

- Protein-rich diets help maintain skin firmness & muscle tone

Conclusion: Reverse Ozempic Face Without Overfilling

Restoring Ozempic Face isn't just about replacing lost fat—it's about strategically rebuilding volume while maintaining natural proportions.

Sculptra & Radiesse for long-term collagen stimulation

HA Fillers for immediate, targeted volume replacement

Skin-tightening treatments to prevent sagging

Preventative maintenance to sustain results

By approaching facial rejuvenation holistically, patients can enjoy weight loss benefits without sacrificing their youthful appearance.

Chapter 56: Fitzpatrick Skin Classification

Why Skin Type Is Not Just About Colour

Understanding the Fitzpatrick Skin Classification is foundational in aesthetic medicine—but it is often misunderstood, oversimplified, or underestimated. Skin tone alone does not determine risk. Genetics, inflammatory response, melanocyte activity, and cultural skin behaviours all play a critical role in how skin reacts to injectables, energy devices, and chemical peels.

This chapter is essential reading for anyone treating skin of colour, mixed-ethnicity patients, or those with a history of pigmentation—even when the skin appears fair.

The Fitzpatrick Skin Types (I–VI)

The Fitzpatrick scale classifies skin based on melanin response to UV exposure, not ethnicity alone.

- Type I – Very fair, always burns, never tans
- Type II – Fair, usually burns, minimal tan
- Type III – Light–medium, sometimes burns, gradually tans
- Type IV – Medium–olive, rarely burns, tans easily
- Type V – Brown skin, very rarely burns
- Type VI – Dark brown to black skin, never burns

Key Clinical Truth

A patient may look Fitzpatrick II or III yet genetically behave like a IV or V when injured or inflamed.

This is where many pigmentation complications occur.

Genetics: Why Fair Skin Can Still Hyperpigment
Skin response is inherited—not just skin colour.

A fair-skinned patient with:

Mediterranean, Middle Eastern,

Asian, Latin, Indigenous or mixed heritage

may carry highly active melanocytes, predisposing them to:

- Post-inflammatory hyperpigmentation (PIH)

- Melasma reactivation

- Prolonged erythema → pigmentation shift

This is why asking about family background matters, even when the skin appears light.

Pigmentation risk is about melanocyte behaviour, not how pale the skin looks on the day of treatment.

Sculptra and Pigmentation Risk (Especially Fitzpatrick IV–VI)

Sculptra is a biostimulatory injectable. It works by creating a controlled inflammatory cascade that stimulates collagen production over time.

Why This Matters for Fitzpatrick V–VI

- Inflammation = melanocyte activation

- Deep or superficial placement errors increase risk

- Nodules or prolonged inflammation raise the likelihood of PIH

Hyperpigmentation after Sculptra is not common, but when it occurs, it is more likely in:

- Fitzpatrick V and VI

- Patients with previous PIH or melasma

- Areas of thin skin or previous trauma

Clinical Pearls

- Use conservative dilution

- Avoid superficial placement

- Meticulous technique and massage education are essential

- Pre-condition high-risk skin when appropriate

The Critical Importance of Fitzpatrick in Chemical Peels

Chemical peels are one of the highest-risk treatments for pigmentation when Fitzpatrick type is ignored.

Higher Fitzpatrick = Higher PIH Risk

Especially with:

- Medium to deep peels

- Overlapping passes

- Inadequate priming

- Poor post-treatment sun avoidance

Safer Peel Strategies for Skin of Colour

- Start low and slow

- Prefer superficial, progressive treatments

- Extend intervals between sessions

- Avoid aggressive endpoints (frosting ≠ success in darker skin)

Pre-treatment skin preparation is non-negotiable for Fitzpatrick IV–VI.

Injectables and Skin of Colour: Specific Considerations

When treating skin of colour, injectors must adapt—not avoid.

Key Differences

- Thicker dermis in many ethnic skins

- Increased fibroblast and melanocyte activity

- Greater risk of visible pigment change after inflammation

Best Practice Principles

- Minimise trauma: fewer entry points, gentle technique

- Avoid unnecessary inflammation

- Respect vascular and anatomical variations

- Avoid treating through active inflammation or acne

Skin of colour does beautifully with injectables—but only when treated intelligently and respectfully.

Post-Inflammatory Hyperpigmentation (PIH)

What Is PIH?

PIH is excess melanin production following:

- Injection trauma

- Heat (energy devices)

- Chemical irritation

- Infection or inflammation

It may appear as:

- Brown, grey, or slate discoloration
- Patchy or localised marks
- Delayed onset (weeks after treatment)

How to Treat PIH (Clinical Overview)

Treatment must be calm, patient, and layered.

Core Principles

- Reduce inflammation
- Suppress melanocyte overactivity
- Support barrier repair
- Protect from UV and heat

Treatment Strategies

- Strict sun protection (daily, non-negotiable)
- Topical pigment regulators (non-irritating)
- Barrier-repair skincare
- Avoid aggressive treatments until pigment stabilises

The worst mistake is "chasing" pigment with more inflammation.
In Fitzpatrick V–VI, patience is not optional—it is the treatment.

Fitzpatrick Is a Safety Tool, Not a Label
The Fitzpatrick classification is not about putting people into boxes—it is about preventing harm.

When respected, it:

- Improves outcomes
- Reduces complications
- Builds trust with patients
- Elevates your clinical skill

CHAPTER 57: BEAUTY ACROSS BORDERS – TREATING FACES FROM AROUND THE WORLD

Understanding Cultural Aesthetics, Ethnic Anatomy, and Global Trends in Cosmetic Injectables

In our increasingly globalized world, aesthetic practitioners must recognize and respect the rich diversity of facial structures, skin types, and cultural ideals of beauty. The "one-size-fits-all" approach is outdated—true artistry lies in enhancing unique features, not erasing them. This chapter explores how different nationalities and ethnic groups perceive beauty and how we can treat their features with skill, cultural sensitivity, and precision.

1. East and Southeast Asians (Chinese, Japanese, Korean, Vietnamese, etc.)

Facial Features:

• Flatter midface

• Wider, shorter nose with a lower nasal bridge

• Smaller eyes with epicanthic folds

• Wider buccal region (cheeks)

• Often smooth and thick dermis with lower pore visibility

Beauty Ideals:

• V-shaped jawline

• High nasal bridge

• Larger eyes with "double eyelids"

• Smooth, clear skin

Popular Treatments:

• Receding Chin Filler and jawline (masseters) thinning with Botox

• Nose bridge augmentation (filler)

• Cheek contouring

• Lip hydration, not volume

• Under-eye filler to address tear troughs

• Eyebrow shaping to lift and widen the eye appearance

2. African and African-American Clients

Facial Features:

• Strong bone structure

• Fuller lips

• Wider nasal base

• Thicker dermis, more melanin (slower aging, but keloid risk)

Beauty Ideals:

• Enhanced, natural cheekbones

• Lip contouring, not reduction

• Skin glow and tone

• Defined jawline

Popular Treatments:

• Sculptra or Radiesse for natural contour

- Lip definition without overfilling

- Hyperpigmentation treatments

- Non-invasive jawline definition

- Botox for brow lift, not flattening expression

3. South Americans (Brazilian, Colombian, Argentinian, etc.)

Facial Features:

- Mixed heritage: Indigenous, European, African

- Strong, diverse bone structure

- Lush lips and expressive features

Beauty Ideals:

- Youthful fullness

- High cheekbones

- Defined lips and sculpted nose

- Glowy, tanned skin

Popular Treatments:

- Cheek enhancement (Voluma, Radiesse)

- Lip filler with a balance of volume and shape

- Botox for smooth skin and brow lift

- PRP or skin boosters for luminosity

4. Western Europeans (French, Spanish, Italian, etc.)

Facial Features:

- Balanced proportions

- Prominent noses (often Roman-style)

- Thinner lips in some regions

- Generally good skin tone

Beauty Ideals:

- Elegant, minimalistic enhancements

- Natural-looking lips

- Defined but soft features

Popular Treatments:

- Lip refinement

- Micro Botox or baby Botox

- Mid-face volume restoration

- Skin tightening without bulk

5. Eastern Europeans (Russian, Ukrainian, Polish, etc.)

Facial Features:

- High cheekbones

- Sharp chin

- Wide-set eyes

- Often paler skin

Beauty Ideals:

- Glamorous, model-like aesthetics

- Plump lips

- Snatched jawline

- Bold cheeks

Popular Treatments:

- Russian lip technique

- Structured cheek filler

- Defined chin and jaw

- Full-face contour packages

6. English (British Isles)

Facial Features:

- Fair skin, prone to redness

- Thin to medium lips

- Lower facial volume in aging

Beauty Ideals:

- Natural enhancement

- Subtle freshness

- Soft lips and eyes

Popular Treatments:

- Baby Botox

- Tear trough filler

- Gentle lip filler

- PRP for skin clarity

7. Americans (USA)

Facial Features:

- Highly diverse (melting pot of ethnicities)

- Media-driven beauty ideals

Beauty Ideals:

- Youthful glow

- Symmetry and proportion

- Plump lips, smooth foreheads

Popular Treatments:

- Full facial rejuvenation (packages)

- Lip filler, cheek and jaw contour

- Skin resurfacing

- Preventative Botox

8. Australians

Facial Features:

- Also diverse—Anglo-Celtic majority but with large Asian, Indigenous, and Mediterranean influences

- Often sun-damaged skin

Beauty Ideals:

- Natural and fresh look

- Subtle tweaks

- Healthy skin focus

Popular Treatments:

- Skin boosters

- PRP and collagen biostimulators

- Lip hydration

- Anti-wrinkle for crow's feet and frown

9. Middle Eastern (Lebanese, Iranian, Arab Peninsula, etc.)

Facial Features:

- Strong nose profile
- Deep-set eyes
- Full lips
- Olive skin tone

Beauty Ideals:

- Sculpted features
- Defined cheeks
- Perfect nose profile
- Sharp brows

Popular Treatments:

- Non-surgical rhinoplasty
- Lip shaping
- Brow lift with threads or Botox
- Cheek contouring

10. India (South Asian Aesthetics)

Facial Features:

- Medium to full lips
- Strong jawline and chin
- Wider midface with well-defined bone structure
- Often high cheekbones and almond-shaped eyes
- Medium to deep skin tones with melanin-rich dermis (slower aging but prone to pigmentation)

Beauty Ideals:

• Smooth, radiant skin

• Symmetrical and softly contoured features

• Refined nose and balanced lips

• Defined jawline and softly lifted cheeks

• Natural expressions with minimal wrinkle lines

Popular Treatments:

• Skin texture and pigmentation improvement (PRP, skin boosters, light peels)

• Subtle lip enhancement—balance and hydrate, not overfill

• Midface volumization to restore youthfulness

• Chin and jawline contouring

• Light Botox for brow lift and expression softening

Trends:

• Natural glam is preferred—results should enhance without drawing attention to the "work"

• Bridal aesthetic is influential: flawless skin, harmonious features

• Increasing interest in collagen biostimulators and thread lifts

Lip Characteristics

Ethnicity/Region	Natural Lip Characteristics	Aesthetic Preferences & Trends	Treatment Approach
English	Thin to medium lips; more definition in the upper lip	Desire for subtle plumpness, symmetry, and hydration	Soft filler for shape and hydration; avoid overfilling
Western European	Moderate fullness; often well-defined shape (e.g., French/Italian)	Favor natural enhancement, soft volume, and proportion	Minimalist techniques with light filler in vermilion border
Eastern European	Naturally fuller lips, particularly lower lip	Bold, structured look; Russian lip technique is popular	Use firm filler, vertical columns for lift and height (e.g., Russian lips)
USA	Highly varied; trend-driven; media influence	Full lips are fashionable; Cupid's bow definition is often emphasized	Contour + volume combo; "Instagram" lips trend with keyhole pout
Asian (East/Southeast)	Evenly proportioned lips; smaller, with less projection	Hydration and shape enhancement, not volume	Use soft filler; focus on cupid's bow and vermilion border
Indian (South Asian)	Medium to full lips; often with good definition and melanin-rich tone	Smoother texture, mild enhancement, and lip symmetry	Focus on lip symmetry, subtle volumizing; balance pigmentation with gloss or hydration
Australia	Diverse population (Anglo, Mediterranean, Asian mix); sun exposure affects texture	Trend toward natural, hydrated lips with mild volume	Balance and blend approach; skin boosters often used alongside filler

Trends by Region

Region	Injecting Trends
East Asia	Chin and jaw slimming with Botox; subtle filler in nose bridge and under-eye areas.
Africa/African-Am.	Cheek sculpting with biostimulators; lip contouring without added volume.
South America	Full facial harmonization; structured filler for cheeks and lips.
Western Europe	Micro-Botox; minimal lip filler; subtle midface rejuvenation.
Eastern Europe	Russian lips; high cheek filler; defined chin and jawline.
UK	Baby Botox; tear trough filler; soft, natural lip enhancement.
USA	Full-face packages; preventative Botox; HD contouring across cheeks and jawline.
Australia	Skin boosters; PRP; conservative filler use to maintain a natural look.
Middle East	Non-surgical rhinoplasty; defined cheekbones; bold lips and brows.
India	Skin texture improvement; subtle lip and midface filler; jawline refinement.

Chapter 58: Reasons Why People Seeking Cosmetic Enhancements

There are many reasons why both women and men seek cosmetic enhancements, and contrary to outdated perceptions, it's often about self-care, confidence, and empowerment—not vanity. Here are some of the key motivations:

1. Career & Professional Image

Age Discrimination in the Workplace: Many professionals feel the pressure to look youthful and energetic to remain competitive, especially in industries that favour younger candidates.

Job Interviews & Promotions: A refreshed, confident appearance can help make a strong first impression.

Public-Facing Roles: Those in client-facing industries—such as sales, hospitality, real estate, and media—often feel the need to maintain a polished image.

2. Social & Personal Confidence

Life after Divorce: A breakup or divorce can lead to self-doubt, and cosmetic enhancements can help rebuild confidence and self-worth.

Dating & Relationships: Looking good often translates to feeling good, which can boost self-esteem when entering the dating scene.

3. Milestone Events

Weddings & Celebrations: Brides, grooms, parents of the couple, and even guests want to look their best for big life events.

Reunions & Social Gatherings: High school reunions, milestone birthdays, or cultural celebrations often motivate people to refresh their look.

4. Everyday Self-Care

Tired-Looking Features: Work stress, lack of sleep, and natural aging can make people look more fatigued than they feel. Treatments like Botox or fillers can help restore a well-rested, refreshed look.

Teachers & Professionals Who Overuse Facial Expressions: Teachers, nurses, and public speakers often develop deep frown lines due to constant expression, making them look stern or tired when they're not.

5. Post-Health Challenges

Weight Loss & Fitness Journeys: Those who have lost weight might seek skin tightening or volume restoration to complement their transformation.

Recovery from Illness: Medical treatments, stress, or chronic illnesses can affect the skin and facial volume, and aesthetic treatments can help restore a sense of normalcy.

6. Men Are Increasingly Seeking Treatments Too

More Men in the Workforce for Longer: Just like women, men also feel the pressure to stay youthful in their careers.

'Tweakments' for a Natural Look: Men prefer subtle treatments to look refreshed without looking "done."

Competition in the Dating Scene: With dating apps and social expectations evolving, men want to maintain an attractive, well-groomed appearance.

Cosmetic enhancement is about self-care, confidence, and feeling good in your own skin, not vanity. Whether it's about career longevity, personal growth, or simply wanting to look as good as you feel, the decision is deeply personal and valid.

Forever Grateful to all my Clients who trust in me, and who have shaped my successful career with their ongoing loyalty.

All my clients have a story.

To be trusted not only with their looks, but with their life story, is a privilege and honour. I have many interesting clients. The role I play within their lives is truly an honour. To assist clients to regain confidence, to witness the events in their lives and in some way be a catalyst for them to have a better life is extremely satisfying. I have always seen myself as the "accidental counsellor"!

One of the many stores in my treasure chest of memories is when a client came to see me for a consultation. As I was taking her before photos, I couldn't help but notice the extreme sadness in her eyes.

• Her face was gaunt.

• Her hair was cut into a simple bob.

• She was thin, with crinkly skin.

• Her lips were tight, as if she were holding back emotions.

She confided in me, her voice trembling:

"My husband left me for a younger woman."

She was devastated.

Determined to regain her confidence, she committed to regular treatments.

• Sculptra to restore volume to her face.

• Fillers to rejuvenate her lips.

• Botox to soften her dynamic lines.

Over the years, her smile grew brighter, her confidence blossomed, and as her outer beauty was restored, her inner glow radiated even more.

Then, karma stepped in.

Eight years later, the younger woman her ex-husband had chosen became obese and neurotic. Meanwhile, my client had transformed like a swan—not only was she beautiful, but her hair had grown into a stylish, flowing look. Her features now carried a quiet confidence, an effortless grace.

At their son's wedding, her ex-husband could not take his eyes off her. His marriage to the younger woman had crumbled, and ten years later, he still regrets leaving her.

But she? She continues to see me every three months, maintaining not just her appearance but her self-assurance and independence.

And he? He lives with regret—while she lives with freedom, beauty, and confidence.

Real Stories from the Treatment Room

What the Needle Has Taught Me

After more than three decades in aesthetic medicine, I've learned that cosmetic treatments are never just about the face. They are about people, emotions, life stages, confidence, heartbreak, reinvention, and sometimes, pure vanity.

The treatment room is a quiet confessional.
Over the years, I've seen women through:

- Marriages

- Divorces

- New relationships

- Illness

- Career changes

- Motherhood

- Menopause

- Reinvention in their 50s, 60s, and beyond

Some of my clients have been with me for decades. I've watched them grow, change, struggle, and flourish. The needle becomes a small part of a much bigger life story.

Here are some of the moments that have stayed with me.

The Tiny Red Dot
One day, a woman in her 50s walked into the clinic.
From across the room, I could see:

- Sun-damaged skin

- Deep frown lines

- Hollow eyes

- Dry, wrinkled texture

In my mind, I was already planning:

- Skin rejuvenation

- Botox

- Possibly some structural support

When I sat her down and asked:
  "What concerns you most?"
She pointed to a tiny red dot on her cheek.
  "That," she said.
It was a small cherry angioma—something that could be easily treated with hyfrecation. She had walked in worried about a tiny red spot, while I was looking at her whole face.

It ws a powerful reminder:
We don't always see ourselves the way others see us.
And as injectors, we must always listen before we treat.

The Loyal Clients
Some clients become part of your life story too.

I've had women who:

- Came to me before their weddings

- Returned after their divorces

- Found new love

- Started new careers

- Became grandmothers

I've watched them grow older, wiser, and often more comfortable in their own skin. We've shared laughter, tears, and countless conversations over the years.

For many, the clinic becomes:

- A safe space

- A place of self-care

- A moment just for themselves

The Overfilled Lips
One young woman came in with:

- Very large, overfilled lips

- Obvious breast implants

- A tiny size 8 body

She sat down and said:
"I want more filler in my lips."
I looked at her carefully and said:
"I think your lips are already overfilled. I'd actually recommend dissolving some of the filler to make them more natural."
She shook her head.
"No. I love the attention they get from men."
In that moment, I realised her lips were not about aesthetics.
They were about validation and attention.
It was not my role to judge her—but it was my role to be honest.
Sometimes, what people want is not what is best for them.

Beauty as a Tool
Another woman came in asking for lip filler.
As we spoke, she told me quite openly that she was a sex worker.
For her, her lips were part of her professional image.
She said:
"My lips are my tools. They're part of how I make a living."
It reminded me again that cosmetic treatments mean very different things to different people. For some, it's confidence. For others, it's identity—or even livelihood.
The Sixty-Year-Old Gentleman

A man in his 60s came in one day, a little nervous but very determined.
He said:
"I've just separated, and I want to start dating again. But I look old and tired next to these younger women."

We discussed subtle treatments:

• Softening his frown

• Improving his skin quality

• A little structural support

A few months later, he returned looking relaxed and confident.

He smiled and said:
"I feel like I've got a second chance."

The Divorced, Sad Woman
One woman came in after a difficult divorce.
She looked exhausted and defeated.
Her concerns were:

• Hollow cheeks

• Deep lines

• Drooping mouth corners

We stated with gentle, staged treatments:

• Botox

• Structural filler

• Skin boosters

Over time, something remarkable happened.

Her face softened.

But more importantly, her energy changed.

She became:

- Brighter

- More social

- More confident

- Independent and happy

The treatments didn't just change her face.

They helped her reclaim herself.

The Cleft Palate Patient
A young woman with a repaired cleft palate came in, very shy and self-conscious about her lips.
With careful, conservative filler, we:

- Balanced her lip shape

- Softened the asymmetry

When she saw herself in the mirror, her eyes filled with tears.
"I've never liked my lips before," she said.
That moment was about far more than aesthetics.
It was about confidence and self-acceptance.

The Woman with Bell's Palsy
A woman who had suffered Bell's palsy came in with a very uneven smile.
Using carefully placed Botox, we:

- Relaxed the stronger side

- Balanced her facial movement

The result was a more symmetrical, natural smile.

She looked at herself and said:
"I feel normal again."
The Girl with No Top Lip
A young woman came in with almost no upper lip.

She felt very self-conscious in photos.
With a small, subtle amount of filler, we:

• Created gentle shape

• Restored balance

The change was not dramatic—but to her, it was everything.

She stood taller, smiled more, and looked far more confident.

The Teacher with the Scary Frown
A schoolteacher came in and said:
"My students are afraid of me. They think I'm always angry."
She had a very deep, permanent frown.
We treated the area with Botox.
When she returned for her review, she said:
"The kids keep asking me why I look so nice lately."
Sometimes, a softened expression can change how the world responds to you.

The Receded Chin and the Wedding Photos
An Asian bride-to-be came in with a very receded chin. She was worried about how she would look in her wedding photos.
With a small amount of chin filler, we:

• Improved her profile

• Balanced her facial proportions

When she saw the result, she smiled and said:
"Now I feel ready for my wedding photos."

Turning Up the Resting Face
One patient complained that she had what she called a "resting bitch face."
Her mouth corners naturally turned downward, giving her a stern expression even when she was relaxed.
With careful treatment:

- Softening the depressor muscles

- Supporting the corners of the mouth

Her expression became softer and friendlier.

She told me later:
   "People smile at me more now."

It Takes All Kinds
One woman with six children came in regularly. Her husband would pay for her treatments and often took her out to beautiful restaurants afterward.
After one full-face rejuvenation, she laughed and said:
   "I suppose I'll have to give my husband a special thank-you on the way home."
Moments like that remind you:
People come from all walks of life, with all kinds of relationships and motivations.
And in this profession, you see it all.

The Tricky Waiting Room
One of the most delicate situations I ever encountered involved a married couple and their company secretary.
The wife came in one day and told me:

- Her husband had an affair with the secretary

- The secretary was manipulative and horrible

Not long after, the secretary also became my client.

She told me:

- The wife was demanding and difficult

- The husband had now moved in with her

The real challenge wasn't the injections.

It was making sure they were never in the waiting room at the same time!

In aesthetics, discretion is everything.

What These Stories Taught Me

Over the years, I've learned that:

- Cosmetic treatments are deeply emotional

- People come for many different reasons

- Confidence can change a life

- Not every request should be granted

- Listening is more important than injecting

But most of all, I've learned this:
The needle is never just about the face.
It is about the person behind it.

And when used with skill, honesty, and compassion, it can do far more than smooth a wrinkle. It can help someone feel like themselves again.

When to Do Aesthetic Treatments, How Often, and How to Plan for Special Occasions

Aesthetic treatments work best when they are timed thoughtfully and planned ahead. While many treatments are described as having "little downtime," the skin and tissues still need time to settle, heal, and look their best.

This section explains when to do each treatment, how often to repeat it, and how far in advance treatments should be performed before an important event.

Planning Around Special Occasions

Whether you are preparing for a wedding, milestone birthday, holiday, professional event, or photo shoot, timing matters.

Even with expert technique, injectables can cause:

- Temporary swelling

- Bruising

- Tenderness

- Asymmetry while settling

General rule:

For injectables, allow at least three weeks before any special occasion.

For first-time treatments or combination treatments, allow four to six weeks.

All you NEEDLE to know:

Last-minute injectables increase stress and reduce control over outcomes.

Botox® / Anti-Wrinkle Treatments

Botox relaxes muscles gradually. Results are not immediate and require time to fully develop.

Botox can be introduced preventatively or used to soften established expression lines.

How often:

Every 3–4 months.

Before a special occasion:

Have Botox performed at least 2–3 weeks before the event.

This allows time for full effect and for any unevenness to be reviewed.

All you NEEDLE to know:

Botox done too close to an event may not have reached its full effect.

Skin Treatments (Non-Injectable)

Skin treatments improve texture, clarity, and glow and support injectable results. Some treatments have minimal downtime, while others cause redness or flaking.

How often:

- Light treatments can be done monthly.

- Corrective treatments are usually performed in courses of three to six sessions.

Before a special occasion:

- Light facials and LED: 3–7 days before

- Peels, microneedling, laser, RF: 3–6 weeks before, depending on intensity

All you NEEDLE to know:

Skin should look calm and settled, not "worked," for important events.

Lip Fillers

Lip fillers can cause swelling and bruising, particularly in the first week. Lips may look uneven while settling.

Lip fillers should be introduced conservatively and reviewed after healing.

How often:

Every 9–18 months.

Before a special occasion:

Allow at least 3–4 weeks.

For first-time lip filler, allow 6 weeks.

All you NEEDLE to know:

Lips need time to soften and integrate — last-minute lips are rarely subtle.

Facial Fillers (Cheeks, Jawline, Chin)

Facial fillers take time to settle into the tissues and for swelling to resolve. Structural fillers should never be rushed.

How often:

Every 12–24 months.

Before a special occasion:

Plan facial fillers 4–6 weeks in advance.

This allows time for bruising to fade and contours to refine naturally.

All you NEEDLE to know:

The face needs time to "find itself" after structural filler.

Biostimulants and Bio-Fillers

Biostimulants do not produce instant results. Their benefit comes from collagen stimulation over time.

How often:

Initial course of one to three treatments, with maintenance every 12–24 months.

Before a special occasion:

These treatments should be done months in advance, not weeks.

They are not event-driven treatments.

All you NEEDLE to know:

Biostimulants are for long-term skin health, not short-term events.

PRP for Face and Neck

PRP can cause swelling, redness, and mild bruising initially. Skin quality improves gradually over weeks.

How often:

Three initial sessions, then maintenance every 6–12 months.

Before a special occasion:

Allow at least 4 weeks after the final PRP session.

All you NEEDLE to know:

PRP enhances glow over time — it is not an instant treatment.

Hands – Radiesse® or Bio-Fillers

Hands may bruise and swell more than the face and require time to settle.

How often:

Every 12–24 months.

Before a special occasion:

Allow 4–6 weeks, especially if hands will be visible in photographs.

All you NEEDLE to know:

Hands reveal bruising easily — timing matters.

When Doing Multiple Treatments

When combining treatments, always work from longest-acting to shortest-acting, and from deep to superficial.

A safe sequence before an event might be:

- Structural fillers and hands first
- Biostimulants well in advance
- PRP
- Botox
- Skin treatments
- Light facials last

All you NEEDLE to know:

Good outcomes are planned, not rushed.

Final Takeaway

All You NEEDLE to Know

Aesthetic treatments are not emergency services.

They are part of a planned, thoughtful approach to ageing well.

If something matters enough to celebrate, it matters enough to plan properly.

When treatments are timed correctly, results look natural, relaxed, and effortless — exactly how good aesthetics should appear.

Disclaimer

This publication is intended as an educational and informational resource, based on the author's personal and professional experiences accumulated over more than three decades in the field of aesthetic medicine and nursing practice.

The content reflects the author's clinical insights, treatment approaches, and interpretations, and does not include formal references or citations to academic literature. It is not intended to replace official training, medical education, or evidence-based clinical guidelines.

Readers are encouraged to exercise professional judgement, refer to current anatomical and pharmacological texts, and comply with local regulations and scope of practice when applying any of the concepts or techniques discussed in this book.

While every effort has been made to present information accurately and responsibly, the author and publisher accept no liability for outcomes resulting from the application of any techniques, interpretations, or procedures described.

This book may include discussion of off-label uses of pharmaceutical products. These are shared from a practitioner perspective for educational purposes only and do not constitute endorsement or medical advice. Additionally, any mention of specific brands or products is intended solely for illustrative purposes; no sponsorship, affiliation, or commercial endorsement is implied.

Nita McHugh is not affiliated with, sponsored by, or endorsing any specific pharmaceutical, skincare, or aesthetic product manufacturers or companies mentioned in this book. All product references are included solely for educational purposes to inform readers about the range of treatments available in cosmetic aesthetics. The content reflects professional experience and is not influenced by commercial interests.

Conclusion

The Artist's Eye: Beyond Points, Protocols, and Perfection

As we reach the end of All You NEEDLE to Know, I invite you to pause—not with your injector's hand, but with your artist's eye.

Because at the heart of everything I've shared in this book—from muscle anatomy to bio-stimulation, from consultation ethics to product science—lies something deeper: the soul of aesthetic medicine is not just knowledge. It is vision.

We begin this journey memorising safe zones and layer depths. We learn where the vessels run, how the ligaments anchor, how light scatters over bone. But the longer we practice, the more we realise: this work is not just technical. It's emotional. It's intuitive. It's human.

You're Not Just an Injector—You're a Storyteller

Every face you treat tells a story. of laughter and grief. of stress and survival. of identity. Your job is not to rewrite that story—it's to honour it.

A cheek isn't just a cheek. It holds memories of joy. A frown line may hold years of resilience. Our goal is never to erase who someone is. It's to illuminate who they are.

Anatomical points give us safety. But artistry gives us grace.

Faces Aren't Templates—They're Landscapes

If there's one lesson I hope stays with you long after the last page, it's this: don't chase dots. Chase balance.

Symmetry is never perfect. Faces are dynamic, expressive, and beautifully unique. One brow lifts a little higher. One eye softens more. One cheek deflates faster than the other. That's real life—and it's your canvas.

When we treat a face holistically, rather than compartmentalised into zones or trends, we create results that feel organic, timeless, and restorative.

Our best work doesn't look "done." It looks right.

Blend, Don't Overfill. Enhance, Don't Inflate.

Natural rejuvenation isn't about chasing volume—it's about managing light and shadow with subtlety. Smooth transitions between planes. Support where there's collapse. Lift where there's heaviness. Glow where skin has dulled.

And above all—restraint.

The injector who knows when to stop is the one who gains trust, loyalty, and long-term success. We are not here to alter faces. We are here to refine them, refresh them, and sometimes—reveal them.

The Future Is Natural. The Future Is You.

There's a rising tide in our industry. A shift back to authenticity. Patients no longer want to look injected—they want to look like the best version of themselves. This is your invitation to evolve with that change. Lead it.

Let your consultations be conversations. Let your needle become an extension of your awareness. Let every treatment plan be bespoke—not just to the face in front of you, but to the soul behind it.

Final Words

You now have all you NEEDLE to know—but what you'll come to understand through experience is this:

- It's not just about the tools—it's how you use them.

- It's not just about the knowledge—it's how you apply it.

- And it's not just about the face—it's how you see.

So go forward—not just as a clinician, but as a compassionate artist.

Inject with skill. Treat with heart.

And remember: the most beautiful results come not from perfection, but from presence.

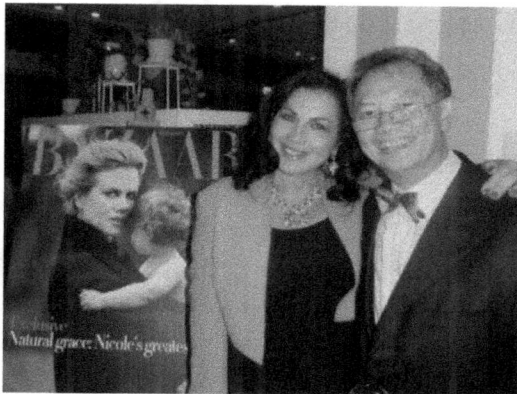

Australian Advanced Aesthetics (AAA)

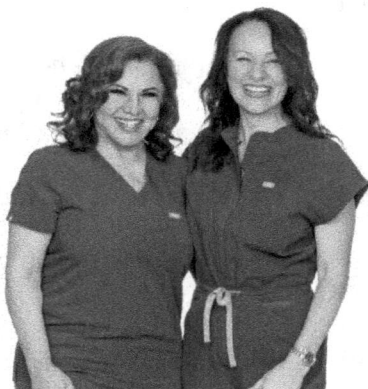

Australian Advanced Aesthetics (AAA) is an educational collective dedicated to advancing excellence, safety, and innovation in cosmetic medicine.

Founded by Dr Bonnie Hawthorne and Registered Nurse Nita McHugh, AAA delivers high-level education through regular hands-on workshops, masterclasses, and immersive aesthetic retreats.

Designed for medical professionals seeking to deepen their clinical knowledge, artistic skill, and confidence, AAA programs focus on evidence-based practice, anatomical precision, patient safety, and ethical aesthetics.

Expressions of interest are welcomed via the official website at www.australianadvancedaesthetics.com.au where upcoming workshops and retreat opportunities are announced.